עת לאהוב

The Newlywed's Guide to Physical Intimacy

עת לאהוב

The Newlywed's Guide
to
Physical Intimacy

JENNIE ROSENFELD, PhD   DAVID S. RIBNER, DSW

Copyright © Jennie Rosenfeld and David S. Ribner
Jerusalem 2011/5771

All rights reserved. No part of this publication may be translated, reproduced, stored in a retrieval system or transmitted, in any form or by any means, electronics, mechanical, photocopying, recording or otherwise, without express written permission from the publishers.

Cover Design: Rami&Jaki
Typesetting: David Yehoshua
Back pamphlet illustrations: Nava Levine-Coren

ISBN: 978-965-229-535-4
3 5 7 9 8 6 4

Gefen Publishing House Ltd.
6 Hatzvi Street
Jerusalem 94386, Israel
972-2-538-0247
orders@gefenpublishing.com

Gefen Books
600 Broadway
Lynbrook, NY 11563, USA
1-800-477-5257
orders@gefenpublishing.com

www.gefenpublishing.com

Printed in Israel   *Send for our free catalogue*

Library of Congress Cataloging-in-Publication Data

Rosenfeld, Jennie.
The newlywed's guide to physical intimacy / Jennie Rosenfeld, David S. Ribner.
  p. cm.
  ISBN 978-965-229-535-4
  1. Intimacy (Psychology) 2. Man-woman relationships.
  3. Newlyweds--Psychology. I. Ribner, David S., 1946- II. Title.
  BF575.I5R65 2011   •   613.9'6--dc23   •   2011020279

Contents

ACKNOWLEDGMENTS / 7

INTRODUCTION / 9

PART 1   THE BASICS / 15

CHAPTER 1   HER BODY/HIS BODY AND AROUSAL / 17
First Impressions 17
The Female Body 19
The Male Body 20

CHAPTER 2   GETTING SEXUAL / 22
Communication – Talking about Sex 23
   We were wondering…
   Talking about Sex before Marriage 25
   Discomfort with Nakedness 26
   Male/Female Gap in Communication 27
Preparing for Your First Sexual Experience 27
Foreplay 29
Kissing 30
Sexual Intercourse 30
   We were wondering…
   Sex Smells 34
   Painful Sex for Wife 34
   Experimenting with New Sexual Activities 35
   New Sexual Position 35
   Not Enjoying Sex 36
Lubrication 37
Female Orgasm 39
   We were wondering…
   No Female Orgasm with Husband 41

Chapter 3   Alternate Intimacies / 42

Oral Stimulation 42
Manual Stimulation 44
  We were wondering…
  Buying Sexual Items 45

Chapter 4   Time as a Factor in Your Intimate Lives / 46

Living with *Niddah*... 46
Pregnancy 48
  We were wondering…
  Sex during Pregnancy... 49
Postpartum 50
  We were wondering…
  Postpartum Sex.. 51
  Baby Interrupting Lovemaking 52

Chapter 5   When Your Sex Life Isn't Working / 54

Men's Concerns 54
  Erectile Dysfunction (ED)... 54
  Rapid or Premature Ejaculation (PE) 55
  Male Orgasmic Disorder (MOD) 55
Women's Concerns... 55
  Vaginismus 55
  Painful Intercourse 56
Concerns for Either Men or Women 56
  Aversion and/or Lack of Interest................................... 56
  Medical Conditions and Medications 57
  Childhood Sexual Abuse 57
  Negative Body Image... 58
  Homosexuality 58
  Pornography 58
  We were wondering…
  Spouse Pressuring Me.. 59
  Working with a Sex Therapist 60

Part 2 Beyond the Basics: Tips and Advice / 63

Chapter 6 She Asks / 65
- Preparing Your Body for the First Sexual Experience 65
- First Sexual Experience – Painful or Not? 66
- No Female Orgasm 67
- No Female Orgasm during Intercourse 68
- *Mikveh* Night Difficulty – Turning Back On 69

Chapter 7 He Asks / 71
- Not Able to Get an Erection 71
- Rapid Ejaculation 72
- *Mikveh* Night Exhaustion 74

Chapter 8 They Ask / 75
- Guilt from Prior Sexual Experiences 75
- Transitioning from No Touch to Full Intercourse 76
- Difficulty with Penetration 77
- Not Ready for Intercourse 78
- Frequency of Sex 79
- Frustration with *Niddah* 80
- Intimacy in Someone Else's Home 82
- External Pressures Affecting Your Sex Life 82

Some Parting Thoughts / 85

Resources / 87
- For Couples 87
- For Women 89
- For Men 90

About the Authors / 92

Acknowledgments

At every step in the creation of this manual, we keenly felt the presence of the *Borei Olam*. We have ventured into sensitive waters and we pray that what we have produced here did not deviate in any way from our obligation to sanctify the Name of Heaven.

While we accept full responsibility for the entire contents of this book, our efforts were aided appreciably by the input of others. Colleagues, friends, and family members willingly shared their comments, suggestions, and criticisms, and we acknowledge here the significance of their contributions (in alphabetical order): Gail Bessler, Shmuel Blitz, Jonathan Feiner, Koby Frances, Joseph C. Kaplan, Peggy J. Kleinplatz, Micki Lavin-Pell, Abby Lerner, Batya Loewenthal, Batsheva Marcus, Chaya Miller, Shoshana Olidort, David Pelcovitz, Ribner family members, Talli Y. Rosenbaum, Pinchas Roth, Alieza Salzberg, Shana Schick, Avi Shmidman, Joseph Telushkin, and Devorah Zlochower.

Thank you to the Metropolitan Council on Jewish Poverty, whose Growth Fund grant given to the Tzelem project in 2007 funded the initial three illustrations that were specially commissioned for this manual. We also wish to express our appreciation to Yeshiva University's Center for the Jewish Future, which, in funding the Tzelem project, sponsored the final two illustrations, and to thank the former Tzelem advisory board members for their support and advice in shaping the initial idea and structure of this manual.

We also wish to thank those individuals who helped fund the publication of this manual.

The team at Gefen Publishing in Jerusalem showed remarkable courage in agreeing to publish this volume. We are indebted to Ilan

Greenfield, publisher; Smadar Belilty, who skillfully guided us through the publication process; and the artful editorial staff.

Finally, this book is dedicated to our families, whose encouragement and understanding gave us the strength to see this project through. We will be forever grateful.

Introduction

As a young couple, you are about to embark on one of life's most important journeys, and we wish you only joy and success. Building a life together can be an immensely satisfying experience, but like any other worthwhile endeavor, it requires an investment from both of you. You have already learned much from your parents and family, teachers, and friends that will help you on your journey. Through this book, we would like to help you navigate this new and uncertain area of your lives: your physical intimacy – the unique pleasure of the sexual experience.

The Creator of the Universe has given you a gift, the ability to enjoy many aspects of your lives – marveling at a beautiful sunset, tasting delicious foods, laughing at a baby's antics. From early on in your lives, you have also experienced the pleasure of a parental hug, kiss, or pat on the back. This background allows you to expect that your initial mutual touch with your spouse will also bring positive feelings. Now that you are a married couple, a much more meaningful experience awaits you.

Your enjoyment as sexual partners is more than just physical; it can bring you to a place of closeness with another person that no other experience can provide. Your sharing of physical intimacy creates an emotional bond that should include feelings of trust, acceptance, caring, and mutuality. Your intimate relationship, which includes your sexual and emotional attachments, is the glue that binds your marriage together.

Shared sexual activity, helped along by hormones, nerve endings, and your five senses, can help you achieve a level of physical pleasure not possible elsewhere in your life. Just keep in mind that no two people are alike regarding sexual feelings and responses, and consequently each of you may experience sexual enjoyment in different ways at different times. As you learn more about yourselves and each other, and develop your own style of communication, you will gain increased insight into the kind of pleasures best suited for each of you. Your physical experiences as a couple go far beyond intercourse itself, and include various intimacies you share during lovemaking and the hugs you give each other at the end of a long day. This joy of discovery can be one of the most gratifying aspects of married life.

We designed this book for use by the *chassan* (groom) and *kallah* (bride), as well as by *chassan* and *kallah* teachers, rabbis, and anyone in the Torah-observant community with questions about sexuality. The language is clear and descriptive, to ensure the accuracy and usefulness of the information. The sexual life of a married couple is a *mitzvah* – one that takes time to learn and is worth the effort to learn well. Regrettably, this area of education has long been neglected in the religious world, and while there has been some recent improvement, no source material of this kind has yet been available.

You may be wondering how Torah-observant Jews can talk about sex in a direct way when it has not been done in the past, and whether the very existence of such a manual might violate the principle of *tzniyus*. This kind of information was once passed from parent to child; our impression is that this is no longer the norm. As a result, many couples are left to face this critical area of their lives with little guidance or information. It is this void we seek to address. Getting the answers you need to important questions will directly influence the quality of your marital relationship.

This book is structured specifically to meet the needs and answer the questions that many observant couples face as they enter marriage and their first years together. Part 1 of the book presents basic sexual information: how your bodies look and work, the basics of sexual behavior, and what to expect as you begin this new phase of your lives. However, many couples will find that this basic knowledge is not enough to respond to a variety of questions and circumstances that may arise. It is for them that we have added the *"We were wondering…"* sections that appear after many topics. The questions and answers in these sections look at specific issues that may challenge couples.

Part 2 of the book – "Beyond the Basics: Tips and Advice" – deals with longer questions and answers. In some cases these questions are specifically oriented to the new couple (such as discussion of wedding-night-related concerns), and in other cases they address issues that emerge over time (such as the frequency of sexual intercourse). What characterizes the second part of the book, aside from the more lengthy question-and-answer format, is that it is focused on giving you practical advice.

You may find that the sections work best when read together, and for this reason we will often refer you to other places in the book where a particular topic is discussed from a different vantage point. Following the page references will allow you to move from part 1 to part 2, getting the answers you need on a particular topic. You may also find the accompaying illustrations helpful, since there may be a limit to what words can explain. Note that all illustrations referenced in the book refer to those in the enclosed envelope in the back.

Just knowing that other couples have grappled with the same issues can provide relief – having doubts in this new area of life is totally expected! Though it is common to face questions and challenges in the sexual realm, especially in the beginning of marriage, some problems would benefit from the guidance of a sexual health professional. If you have been working on a problem on your own for a while and the situation is not improving, it never hurts to ask. The information and suggestions below are not intended as a substitute for therapy or for a necessary medical intervention. Take a look at chapter 5, "When Your Sex Life Isn't Working," if you think your issue might require therapy or medical treatment.

This book is far from exhaustive. Many helpful and more specific works have been written on different aspects of sexuality; at the end of this book you will find a list of resources, should you desire further information. Some topics related to sexuality – specifically conception, fertility, and birth control – are not within the scope of this volume. If you need information in these areas, your first stop should be your doctor.

Some notes of caution: though this manual is written to ease the transition to marriage for Torah-observant couples, this is not a work of *halachah*. We hope couples will find that the language, diagrams, and range of issues make this manual more comfortable to use than generic sex manuals; however, we have designed it to be used by a wide range of Torah-observant Jews who follow a range of halachic opinions. So, if any part of this booklet raises religious questions for you, we urge you to ask a rabbinic authority who knows you as a couple and who is well versed in this area of Jewish law.

You may also find that there are parts of this book that don't speak to you for one reason or another – some information might be too basic, and other information might be beyond your current comfort zone. It is a complex task to write a book on such sensitive subject matter that is meant to address a wide constituency. While we have done our best, there will probably be parts of this manual that are not relevant for you, so just skip them!

A word may be in order about who we are and why we have decided to write this book. We are both Torah-observant Jews who have been involved with issues of sexuality in the Orthodox and ultra-Orthodox community. One of us has worked as a sex therapist in this community for over thirty years and has seen hundreds of couples with sexual problems, and one of us has worked on communal consciousness-raising and sexual education for only a few years. However, both of us have seen couples and individuals whose sexual lives could have been enhanced and whose problems could have been prevented with adequate education and information. We have seen people who felt alone and isolated for harboring feelings and desires that were completely normal, and others who were unfamiliar with their own sexuality and hesitant to establish deep sexual connections with their spouses. We have seen people who have had difficulty making the transition from the unrealistic sexuality of the media to the real-life sexuality of marriage. And it is for these reasons that we decided to write this manual.

Sexuality is a beautiful part of life – truly a gift from God – and we hope that as young couples beginning this journey, you have the mutual trust to be open with each other, to enjoy your sexuality and make it a meaningful part of your relationship. Sexuality at its best is a holistic experience involving body and soul and a range of emotions, and we hope that as a couple you find that range of sexual connections to sustain and nourish you throughout your lives.

We join your family and friends with the blessing that you merit

"ששון ושמחה... גילה רינה, דיצה וחדוה, אהבה ואחוה, ושלום ורעות."

"…joy and gladness… mirth, song, delight and rejoicing, love and harmony, and peace and companionship."

Mazal tov!

Part 1
The Basics

Chapter 1

Her Body/His Body and Arousal

Before discussing sexual activity, it is important to have a clear understanding of how your bodies react to sexual messages and get ready for intimate physical contact. While sexual contacts go beyond the physical and encompass a range of emotions, it is essential that you know enough about your own body and your spouse's body to allow for a comfortable and pleasurable sexual experience. What follow are the basics; for more in-depth information, see some suggestions in the resources section.

First Impressions

It may seem obvious, but it is important to stress that no two bodies are exactly alike – each person's body looks different from any other and each may respond differently to the same types of stimulation. While you may have certain expectations about the ideal appearance, your spouse's body will likely look different than you might imagine.

In contrast to a woman's body, much of the male body is generally covered with hair. The male body is also shaped differently than the female body: the male torso is generally shaped like an upside-down triangle, widest at the shoulders and narrower at the hips, while the female torso is shaped like a pear, narrower on top and wider at the hips, and more curvaceous than the male body. Body weight is distributed differently in each sex, so be prepared not to face your mirror image when you see your spouse without clothing.

In terms of the female body, one surprise is how much it changes: life-cycle events, such as pregnancy and nursing (more about these on pages 48–53) change a woman's body shape, as well as possibly affecting her sexual interest level. One organ that is different in the male and female bodies is the breasts, which for many women are considered an erogenous zone (a part of the body whose stimulation is likely to produce sexual arousal). Breast size varies widely from one woman to another and even for the same woman over the course of her life. As with penis size (and the size of any other body part), the size of a woman's breasts doesn't affect her sexual functioning or enjoyment.

These differences – and the opportunity now awaiting you to learn about and explore your spouse's body – can be a source of great excitement. Take your intimate relationship slowly; take the time to discover the uniqueness of your spouse's body, his or her distinctive physical features, and his or her response to your touch.

Skin-to-skin contact can be intensely erotic; through touching and exploring your spouse's whole body, you will learn how and where to caress in order to share the most pleasure. This exploration can be an ongoing part of your shared intimacy. While certain parts of the body are known as erogenous zones, areas especially sensitive to sexual stimulation, the whole body is well worth exploring. You will find that when you massage or caress certain areas, your spouse may respond in one of several ways. In general, the touch may be experienced as positive, neutral, sexually arousing, or negative. Be guided by your spouse's response.

Erogenous zones include the breasts, nipples, buttocks, and genitals. However, each individual has his or her own sexual preferences, so you may find that for you or your spouse a touch on the nape of the neck, or behind the ear, or the palm of the hand can engender an intimate feeling. You may also find that mindset is important: we are human beings and not machines, so stimulating your spouse's erogenous zones is not like pushing a button that leads to an automatic response. You will likely find that stimulation only works when you or your spouse are emotionally open to being stimulated. Only through openness and exploration will you learn about what gives your spouse the most pleasure. So have fun and explore!

The Female Body

The envelope at the back of the book contains labeled illustrations of both the male and female genitals. Below, we will describe the sexual organs of each gender. Be aware that your genitals as well as those of your spouse won't look exactly like the ones in the diagrams, though they will contain the same anatomical parts.

Take a look at illustration 1; you will see a woman's external vaginal area (known as the *vulva*), viewed as if she were lying on her back, with her legs apart. Three openings are visible. The first, the urethra, allows for urination, and the third, the anal opening, allows for bowel movements. The second or middle opening is the vaginal opening, which is where you insert a tampon, do a *bedikah*, and where the penis enters in an action called *penetration*. Surrounding the vaginal opening are two layers of lips, and above this opening is a small piece of tissue called the *clitoris*; to find the exact location of the clitoris, follow the inner lips to where they meet together on top.

The entire area of the vulva, inside and out, is full of nerve endings, making it very sensitive to touch, thus allowing for pleasurable feelings when it is caressed in a manner comfortable for each woman. The clitoris in particular has myriad nerve endings, requiring an especially gentle touch, but also providing a trigger for the intense sexual response called an *orgasm*. The right kind and length of clitoral stimulation varies from woman to woman, so it is important that each bride, through her exploration of her vulvar area, either alone or with her husband, gets to know the kind of caress most enjoyable to her so she can teach it to her husband.

When a woman experiences physical or emotional sexual feelings, her body may respond in different ways, the result of various hormonal changes. One type of response is the production of vaginal *lubrication*. Lubrication is a liquid substance produced in the vagina, usually the result of being aroused in some way, such as by kissing or caressing. This kind of arousal sends a message to her brain to prepare for sexual intercourse, and one response is to enable the vagina to accept an erect penis in as smooth a way as possible. Thus this lubrication acts to reduce the likelihood of painful penetration and to enhance the experience of intercourse.

For many women who want to be intimate with their husbands, sufficient natural lubrication accumulates in the vagina. When, for whatever reason, this process does not produce adequate lubrication for comfortable penetration and *thrusting* (movement of the penis within the vagina), several types of artificial lubrication are available for purchase. Especially during the initial sexual experiences (when women may experience insufficient lubrication), it can be helpful to have a lubricant available. We discuss lubrication more fully on pages 37–39.

As sexual arousal builds and stimulation continues, a woman will generally reach the phase of *orgasm*. An *orgasm* is a series of contractions of the muscles surrounding the vagina, which produce an intense feeling of pleasure and warmth. Even after orgasm, many women will be amenable to further stimulation. (In the next section, we discuss the place of orgasm in the process of sexual intercourse.)

The Male Body

Illustration 2 shows a man's circumcised penis. The long part or shaft consists of a tube in the middle running from inside his body to the opening at the end, called the urethra. Most of the time, this is used to pass urine from the body. During sexual intercourse, this is the tube that will direct semen, containing sperm, into her vagina. The scrotum is a skin sack containing the testes, two oval glands that produce sperm. The shaft is made up of sponge-like material and is entirely covered by skin also containing many nerve endings, which provide a pleasurable feeling when touched. For most men, the top of the penis is the most sensitive area. Unlike the vagina, the penis is a dry organ that has no scent.

The dotted lines show roughly what a penis looks like when it is hard or *erect*. When a man becomes sexually interested or aroused, a biochemical response allows for more blood than usual to flow into the penis, which fills the sponge-like material, resulting in an erection. This hardness is necessary for smooth penetration into the vagina during intercourse. For the new *kallah*, seeing her husband's erect penis can be confusing; the penis, which in its relaxed state is about 1–2 inches long and the color of the rest of his skin, enlarges to about three times that size. When erect, the penis can become a deep red and almost purple as his arousal increases, with veins along the penis becoming more pronounced, and pre-seminal fluid sometimes dripping out (this is not semen, although it may contain a small number of sperm cells). These changes are normal and should not be a cause of concern.

The average length of an erect penis is about 5–6 inches (though penis size varies), but just about any length can easily fit into her vagina, which can hold it snugly enough to provide enjoyment for both of you during penetration and thrusting. For him, the result of this thrusting is increased feelings of physical pleasure in the penis, leading to the intense experience of orgasm. Orgasm is the rhythmic contraction of muscles near the base of his penis that pump sperm into the vagina. Once the orgasm is completed, his penis will return to its relaxed state. For a period afterwards, known as the *refractory period*, he will be unable to achieve another erection even when stimulated; this time period varies from man to man, and even for the same man over the course of a lifetime.

Chapter 2

Getting Sexual

In this section we explain some of the specifics of sexual intercourse. As you read through these paragraphs, we ask that you keep in mind several general guidelines:

- You should expect your initial sexual activities together to be a learning experience; give yourselves the time and patience to grow with each other in this new realm of interaction.

- Sex for you may not be like anything you've seen or heard from movies, books, or friends. These and similar sources may create unrealistic expectations that sex is never awkward, proceeds naturally without obstacles, and is always enjoyable from the first time onward. In reality, men do not enjoy sex more than women, things do not have to happen spontaneously, and both of you need to take responsibility for making your sex life work.

- Sex should be fun and enjoyable in whatever way you feel comfortable, but until you get a clearer sense of what this means to each of you, the process of discovery should be a shared and eagerly anticipated journey.

- Men and women tend to differ regarding almost every aspect of sex and intimacy. This means that if the two of you are together sexually, you may both find the experience to be truly enjoyable, but each of you may enjoy it in different ways – she may look forward more to the closeness and warmth, he may desire the physical intensity (or vice versa). In addition, you may each respond differently to exhaustion, worry, or a visit from your parents. You can avoid much frustration and misunderstanding by not expecting your husband or wife to see things as you do and by clearly communicating your own sexual needs and expectations.

+ If your intimate life just isn't working, don't hesitate to get professional help. One word about seeking a therapist, in case it's something you haven't done before: Speaking to a therapist when a problem arises is not worth obsessing over. You wouldn't hesitate to go to a doctor if you broke your leg or were dealing with some other physical ailment; likewise, going to a therapist is just something you should do when you realize that you're experiencing a problem of this nature. Oftentimes, if you catch a problem early and try to deal with it as soon as possible, it will be more quickly treatable than if you wait until the problem escalates.

Communication – Talking about Sex

Being sexual with each other is a unique form of communication, but that experience can be made more secure and comfortable if your verbal communication – what you each say and hear – conveys clear messages. You have accumulated many years of experience talking about things you know and for which your conversation flows smoothly: to ask and answer, to request and explain, to bring joy and express anger. Now, as you enter a world of unfamiliar human behavior, a new communication challenge awaits you.

In this section we will be emphasizing the importance of verbal communication. For those couples, however, for whom talking openly about sex may be uncomfortable (or even considered improper conduct), the guidelines that follow should help determine which kinds of nonverbal communication (gestures, caresses, guiding your spouse's hands) provide the clearest messages.

As a first step, it is important that you become familiar and at ease with the names of the *parts of your bodies* associated with sexual activities, such as vagina, penis, breasts, nipples, clitoris. Whether you use this formal language, alternate terms heard elsewhere, or create words of your own (as some couples do), you both should support each other's attempts to find the easiest, clearest, and most comfortable ways to describe your bodies.

The next step is to learn the terms that indicate sexual responses and activities. If you have read this far, you now are familiar with words such as sexual intercourse, lubrication, erection, penetration, thrusting, and so on. If you are uncomfortable expressing these terms verbally, you might try practicing them aloud when you are by yourself, then say them to each other at a relaxed time. You may blush or giggle and that's just fine; this is new for both of you, so share this piece of learning together. The better the atmosphere between you, the quicker you will overcome your hesitations.

The final, and often most difficult, step is learning to talk about your feelings, such as desires, fears, expectations, and fantasies. During the first months of your marriage, talk with each other about your hesitations and anxieties. No one expects either of you to be a sexual expert; verbally sharing the newness of this experience gives you a partner – neither of you should feel alone. Try not to make the mistake of assuming your husband or wife knows what is on your mind without your having expressed yourself in words. No one is telepathic, and counting on your intuition often leads to painful misunderstandings; as difficult as it may be, it is critical that each of you learn to express your own sexual needs to each other. Learning to be aware of your preferences and to articulate them will help bring you closer as a couple and give you a more positive and fulfilling sexual relationship. To ensure that your messages are heard, learn to express yourselves clearly and to listen carefully. Be aware that this experience is new for both of you and feelings can be hurt easily.

As you become more at ease with each other, you may wish to consider adding additional options to your sexual activities (a different sexual position, for example) or sharing sexual fantasies with each other (such as being together on a deserted beach). Two points are important here:

- You should work toward feeling sufficiently comfortable to express and hear any sexual request that either of you finds of interest.
- You both have the right to say no to anything you do not wish to do.

The right to say no is basic to the trust you will build with each other, but equally important is knowing *how* to say no. To avoid causing feelings of rejection, try to ensure that after saying no, you offer an alternative sexual activity or time to be together: "I'd rather not do this, but I'd love to do that with you," or "This is not a good time for me, but let's make a date for tomorrow night." Adding some words of affection will also go a long way toward enhancing your feelings of intimacy.

We were wondering...

Talking about Sex before Marriage

THEY ASK: We've been engaged for more then a month now and have a very open style of verbal communication along with a strong commitment to being shomer negi'ah *until our marriage. We've always felt like we can talk about anything with each other, though lately this has led us into detailed sexual conversations about our desires, fantasies, and fears. Is it wrong to talk about sex during engagement? Sometimes it feels not* tzanu'a, *but on the other hand*

> *we want to walk into marriage feeling comfortable and ready for sex... What should we do?*

The fact that you're able to talk so openly is a great sign, as good communication is probably the most important factor in ensuring a good marriage and a positive sexual relationship. Before getting married, it's important to talk about your emotions and fears concerning sexuality, so that you can begin your marriage with a sense of each other's feelings. However, if you want to continue being *shomer negi'ah* until your wedding, there's no need to get specific about fantasies and actions at this point.

Discomfort with Nakedness

> *The issue of being naked is really bothering me – I am really nervous that my spouse won't like the way I look naked and that I won't like the way my spouse looks naked either, and I'm also scared to be completely naked with my spouse so soon after we get married... Help!*

It's okay to feel anxiety and it can help to discuss that emotion with your spouse, who may just feel the same way! Take things slowly and at a pace that allows you to feel comfortable. You might want to remove some of each other's clothing (as much as you feel comfortable with) and then remove the rest when you're under the covers. You're probably both feeling unsure of yourselves, and having your initial experiences of being naked with each other under the covers can feel a lot less threatening. Like anything new, feeling comfortable being naked with your spouse takes time, and for most couples, this period of awkwardness passes quickly.

> **MALE/FEMALE GAP IN COMMUNICATION**
>
> *THEY ASK: As we have become more comfortable talking with each other about sex, we realize that we often look at sex very differently and sometimes that difference causes painful moments and misunderstandings. What should we do?*
>
> It's true that you are different in many ways, and not just physically. However, realizing that men and women can sometimes differ in just about every aspect of their sexuality can prevent some difficult times. One example of this female/male difference frequently occurs when you desire to be together at the end of a busy day. For most men, this means that almost everything else becomes less important than starting and completing whatever sexual activity the couple wishes. Women, however, tend to be more connected to the world around them, and unless they feel comfortable in their environment, sex may not be at the top of their list. Thus if she says she cannot get into bed and truly feel relaxed until the dishes are done, he will be able to anticipate this in the future and know to help so that they can both feel comfortable about getting sexual.

Preparing for Your First Sexual Experience

After the intense experience of all that leads up to standing together under the *chuppah*, you will have a brief period of time to spend with each other before greeting your family and friends. There are no rules about what to do in the *yichud* room, but in addition to ending their fast, couples tend to use this time to experience some initial mutual touch. Because of time and place constraints, this is usually limited to holding hands, a hug, and a kiss. Sometimes, to minimize the uncertainty of this moment, the *chassan* will place a bracelet or necklace on the *kallah*.

For couples who have had no prior physical contact, these moments may be awkward and uncertain. You are not alone. Not only is this a new experience, it occurs during a time of intense emotions. Take a slow, gentle approach, being sensitive to how nervous you or your partner may be. Because every couple's experience will be different, there are no objective expectations. If you can also laugh a bit with each other, you will leave the *yichud* room ready to celebrate at your *simchah*.

The first time you actually have sexual intercourse presents some unique challenges. *When* to attempt penetration should be a topic you discuss with each other. You may have the desire and the energy to consummate your marriage (that is, to have sexual intercourse) that first night, and if both of you feel that way, there is no reason to wait. You may, however, find yourselves too exhausted on your first night together to do more than hold hands and share some hugs and kisses. Some couples may even decide together to wait a few nights and get more comfortable with one another before attempting intercourse. A good night's sleep can do wonders to increase your comfort level as you look toward your first sexual experience as a married couple.

To get ready physically, start with a shower and brush your teeth. If perfume, cologne, or aftershave makes you feel good, then put some on. In choosing what to wear, the first rule is to disregard any well-meaning advice from friends and relatives and be guided by what makes you feel comfortable and desirable; the better you feel about yourself, the more satisfying this experience will be. It is what you say and how you act that makes up the message you wish to convey to your spouse, not only the way you dress.

To prepare emotionally, remember you have been blessed with the ability to have physical enjoyment. Even though the first few times may be awkward, a bit scary, and sometimes uncomfortable, you are building a mutual experience that will hopefully last the lifetime of your marriage. These intimate moments can significantly enhance your relationship as can no other aspect of your lives together.

For some couples, the anxiety, uncertainty, or awkwardness they feel as they think about their initial sexual connection may cause a more extended delay in attempting intercourse. Be patient with each other and share your feelings; sometimes just talking about it can ease the tension.

No matter how much theoretical information you have in advance, actually having sexual intercourse can only be learned by doing. Your first attempts may seem clumsy and not entirely enjoyable; if so, you are like just about everyone else. Don't lose hope and faith in each other. Keep at it; the more you practice, the more sex becomes comfortable and a source of mutual pleasure.

Foreplay

The word "foreplay" refers to various kinds of intimate touch that a couple can enjoy with each other before they have actual sexual intercourse (see pages 30–33). There are no specific guidelines that define foreplay, and the range of possibilities is entirely up to each couple's comfort level. In general, couples make use of foreplay to gradually enhance their sexual activity, starting with less intense touches such as a back massage and then progressing to more specifically sexual and intense activities.

We will offer some limited suggestions for foreplay activities, but we want to emphasize that couples should feel free to explore on their own various ways to touch each other and provide mutual pleasure before they move on to intercourse. Be guided by your partner's response; the clearer your communication, the more you can be certain of pleasing each other. There is no ideal amount of time for foreplay, but the longer you both can engage in these activities, the longer you can enjoy your time together.

Among the gentler and less intense foreplay activities are handholding, hugs, gentle kissing, and non-genital massages. Moving on, you can try taking off your own or each other's clothing, hugging each other without any clothing, more intense kissing, gentle breast or genital touch, bathing together, or massages with creams or oils. More intensely sexual activities may be nipple and breast stimulation – with fingers or lips and tongue – and more direct genital touch.

Kissing

Kissing is one of the most intimate of human activities. For almost all of us, it is part of our lives from our earliest moments and it continues to be an ongoing aspect of various relationships – for example, kissing our parents and children. In an intimate marital relationship, kissing can convey many different messages: *good morning, have a great day, happy birthday, sleep well*, and, of course, *I love you*.

Learning how to kiss each other should be enjoyable for both of you. Here we offer you a few guidelines to start you in the right direction. Make sure that your first experiences are gentle. Lips come with many nerve endings, which allow for the positive feelings of kissing but which can also bruise easily. So start with some light kisses on cheeks, forehead, ears, and neck (the order is up to you); then move to similar kisses on closed lips. Talk with each other about how this feels, what each of you liked and did not like.

Kisses on any other area of your body may also be enjoyable and may become part of your foreplay. Go slowly, making sure that each of you is comfortable with the body location and intensity of these kisses. You might want to try starting with some kisses at one side of the base of the neck, kissing slowly up across each other's lips, then down to the base of the neck on the other side.

Some people enjoy using their tongues to give and receive kisses. If you would like to give this a try, remember that your tongue is not a battering ram; start off with some gentle tongue touches on each other's lips, then talk with each other about what you might like to do next.

Sexual Intercourse

For many couples, the most intense and enjoyable aspect of sexual activity is what is known as sexual intercourse. Take a look at illustration 3, which shows sexual intercourse, or the entry of a man's penis into a woman's vagina. This should happen after foreplay when the man's penis is erect and the woman's vagina is lubricated. Erection and lubrication usually result from both of you feeling excited to be with each other sexually and from the foreplay activities, such as caressing and stroking each other's erogenous zones. His erection, which indicates his readiness for intercourse, will be obvious. However, because lubrication is internal, it would be helpful if either of you could gently insert a finger in her vagina to check whether it is wet (if you feel comfortable with this). In addition, it is crucial to check in with each other and see if you each feel ready to proceed. Ask your wife whether she feels ready for sexual intercourse, as vaginal lubrication does not always serve to indicate emotional readiness. See pages 37–39 for more on lubrication.

Because your sexual organs are covered with thousands of nerve endings, intercourse can become an intensely pleasurable experience, connecting you both physically and emotionally. Don't worry if it takes some months to really enjoy intercourse; spend as much time as you need just getting comfortable with each other. Your bodies are designed to allow penetration to happen with ease, but no two bodies are exactly the same. No matter how much you know theoretically about how men and women are built, your husband or wife is different from any other person on the planet, so fitting together sexually may take you some time to figure out. This is done most easily with patience, gentleness, and understanding. Should any kind of vaginal touch lead to recurring pain, please be aware that this is a correctable condition; see pages 55–56 where we deal more with this issue. Though the first few times may be awkward or uncomfortable, sexual intercourse can become a fun and connecting part of your lives as well as a deeply spiritual experience.

Illustration 3 shows you how to position your bodies in the manner that is used most often around the world. The woman should position herself first, lying on her back, feet flat on the bed, knees bent and raised, legs spread apart as comfortably as possible. It may also be more comfortable if a pillow is placed under her buttocks. The man is partially on his knees between her legs, with his hands or elbows and arms on either side of his wife. He then moves his hips forward so that his penis can enter her vagina, an action called *penetration*. To ensure that his penis gets to the right place, the woman may need to hold her husband's penis and give it some guidance.

Once you have successfully made this connection, the man should move his hips so that his penis moves forward and backward inside her vagina, without its coming out altogether. These motions are called *thrusting* and should increase the pleasure of this activity. As with all aspects of sexual intercourse, expect this to take some time to get used to. While this thrusting takes place, the woman can move her hips in the same rhythm as her husband's movements, further enhancing the experience. She also has her hands free to caress her husband as she may wish.

These thrusting motions should be started gently, with the option of varying the pace as you both desire; just make sure that whatever you do is acceptable to each of you. Your genital areas are sensitive, so too hard or rapid a motion may be painful. As you become more comfortable with each other, you may also try varying the depth of penetration.

Thrusting generally stops after the man reaches orgasm and ejaculates. This occurs as a result of the stimulation to his penis during the thrusting motions. At this point, his penis usually loses its hardness and slips out of her vagina, although if he remains erect he can continue thrusting. While most men reach orgasm as a result of intercourse, many women do not, simply because they do not experience sufficient clitoral stimulation through this kind of physical touch. So it is possible that once the husband reaches orgasm, he will feel a sense of satisfaction, while his wife remains aroused and desirous of further stimulation to help her reach orgasm. In this situation, if the woman is close to reaching orgasm, he can ask her if she would like him to continue stimulating her clitoris and/or vagina until she reaches orgasm.

Another possibility is for the husband to focus on pleasuring his wife and giving her an orgasm *before* as well as during or after penetration. As we have explained earlier, most women are able to reach orgasm through clitoral stimulation, and as you have seen in illustration 1, the clitoris is located slightly above the vaginal opening. Part of learning about your bodies is discovering the kind of clitoral touch best suited to bring your wife maximum sexual pleasure. Depending on each spouse's comfort level, the husband may wish to use one or two fingers to caress the lips surrounding the vagina, to slowly insert his finger into the vaginal opening, or to gently stimulate the clitoris. He should be guided by the kind of touch that brings his wife maximum pleasure; clear communication is especially important.

Generally speaking, mutual satisfaction is the goal of each sexual encounter, with each of you defining your own personal pleasure. It is of particular importance that neither of you assume that the kind of sexual enjoyment you want is exactly what your partner wants. The ability of each of you to be sensitive to and understanding of the other stands at the heart of true sexual union, physically and emotionally.

After the intensity of sexual intercourse, you may be feeling especially close to each other. To maintain this feeling, stay with each other in bed for a while, using gentle hugs and caresses to enhance your intimate feelings. If either of you wishes to wash yourself right after intercourse, feel free to do so; then you can get back into bed and sleep the night together.

After intercourse, you may feel or notice a wet spot on the sheets. This "mess" is a normal part of sex and is the result of some of her lubrication dripping out of her vagina, along with some of his semen. Laundering will take care of the spot; some couples place a towel on the bed before intercourse, to minimize the laundry hassle. Women who are bothered by the wet spot on their underwear the next day can wear a mini-pad or panty-liner to absorb the moisture.

We were wondering...

Sex Smells

SHE ASKS: We've been married for around six weeks and due to niddah we've only had intercourse twice so far. However, I've noticed each time that I smell weird after sex. Is there something wrong with me or is this normal?

Welcome to the world of being sexually active – sex comes with its own unique smells, noises, and messiness, and you'll soon get used to them and find your own ways of coping. While the smell might seem like a big deal, you are most likely the only person who notices it, so don't worry; if it truly bothers you, you can easily take care of it by showering after intercourse. Some women also find that their bodies make certain sounds during sex (such as a swishing sound from the wetness of lubrication of the vagina, or the sound of passing wind), and these noises are also normal. These things can feel strange, but just keep in mind that right now you're at the very beginning of working out your sexual relationship and everything is new, but with time you'll become more comfortable.

Painful Sex for Wife

HE ASKS: We got married a few months ago, and whenever I have sex with my wife she experiences a lot of pain. Her hymen broke the first time we were together, and there is no more bleeding, but every time I penetrate she suffers. It does get a little better once I am inside, but she is getting almost no pleasure from it, and she just wants it to be over. We've been using a lot of artificial lubrication, as we were instructed to, but it just doesn't seem to help. What can we do?

Pain during intercourse is something that most women will experience at some point in their lives. However, sex is not supposed to hurt. It is a sign that something is not quite right and requires attention. The good news is that it is easily treatable and that in cases like this the root of the pain is almost always physical and not emotional. It seems that you've done the best you can, and now might be the time to see a doctor or physical therapist who specializes in treating painful sex.

Experimenting with New Sexual Activities

THEY ASK: We've been married for over a year, and while our sexual life had been pretty routine until now (we were still just trying to figure things out), we recently started to try something new. It's not something we've seen in a book or anything like that, and we're just wondering whether that's normal.

If whatever you're doing is something that both of you desire, then it's great that you feel comfortable enough to be creative in your sexual life. Just be sure that before trying anything new you communicate openly with each other to determine that both of you are comfortable – if so, then enjoy!

New Sexual Position

HE ASKS: We've been married for around a year, and lately my wife has begun to hint to me that we should try a new sexual position. I don't really feel comfortable with this, and I don't know how to tell her.

If your wife is suggesting something that you don't feel comfortable with, you don't have to do it. The best option is to have an open conversation where you can make clear how you feel about trying a new position. It may be helpful to find out why your wife is interested in another position – perhaps your usual sexual position is causing her pain or isn't allowing her to have an orgasm. If so, you can try some of the suggestions on pages 39–41 to better understand each other's needs and ultimately deepen your sexual relationship. Perhaps she is feeling uncomfortable with too much of your body weight leaning on her in the man-on-top position. Perhaps she just wants to try something new. If so, talk about something new that you would both feel comfortable trying. Having an open conversation can help you both.

Not Enjoying Sex

SHE ASKS: We've been married for nearly a year, and though I feel that we've mastered the mechanics of having sex, and I'm not feeling any pain, I'm not feeling any pleasure either.

There are a few things that may be going on here. To start with the simplest, if the issue is that you're unable to reach orgasm through intercourse, then take a look at pages 39–41 and 67–69, which talk more about female orgasm and suggestions for how to make it happen (either on your own or in the context of intercourse).

However, if lack of orgasm isn't your issue, or isn't your only issue, then this may be something that you should be talking to a professional about. If what you're feeling is something along the lines of "I love my husband, but I'm just not able to make love to him," or "I love my husband, and I can do the physical parts of sex, but I'm just not feeling any enjoyment," then seeking out a sexual health professional is the right step to take. See pages 60–61 for more about seeing a therapist.

Lubrication

Adequate lubrication is essential for comfortable penetration and a mutually pleasurable sexual experience. While artificial lubrication may not be necessary for you, for some couples using a lubricant will make sex more comfortable, especially the first few times they engage in intercourse.

The concept behind using a lubricant is that the vaginal tract needs to be wet in order for the penis to enter comfortably, and for the sexual experience to feel pleasurable for both husband and wife. A woman's body, when aroused, usually produces this lubricant naturally. However, for the first few attempts at intercourse, when the woman is still getting used to the newness of sex, and at other times during a woman's life cycle, this natural lubrication may not occur as quickly or at all. Therefore, using a store-bought lubricant can ease the discomfort of dry sex. The lubricant should be applied according to the instructions on the package, and applying it can become part of your foreplay.

One note of caution: natural vaginal lubrication is a tricky area, being in some – but not all – cases the woman's physical sign that she is ready for penetration. One should never use artificial lubrication as a substitute for the wife's arousal, just as natural lubrication alone should not be taken as an absolute indicator of her arousal. To be clear, while lubrication shows that a woman is physically ready for sex, it doesn't say anything about whether she is psychologically and emotionally in the mood, so don't take lubrication as a substitute for communication!

Some women produce more lubrication than others, and the amount of lubrication changes at different times during a woman's menstrual cycle and during different stages of a woman's life. Women who are nursing may lubricate less, as well as those taking medications such as birth control pills, or those dealing with other medical conditions.

Often young couples hear about only one type of lubricant – KY Jelly – however, many other options are available and may be more user-friendly. Depending on where you live and where you are shopping, there are about as many varieties and different brands of lubricant as there are cereals. Since brands vary so widely, here are a few general principles that you can keep in mind when looking for a lubricant:

- Saliva is by far the best lubricant.

- In second place are olive oil and almond oil (and any other natural oil). However, watch out for the expiration dates and make sure you're not using oil that has spoiled (because a little lubricant goes a long way, a one-liter container can take a long time to finish!).

- Don't confuse oil with Vaseline, petroleum, or any other mineral oil, as these can irritate a woman's vagina. A regular massage oil should not generally be used for intercourse, unless the package indicates that it is safe for penetration.

- In choosing commercial lubricants, you have several different options that each have their pros and cons:
    - Water-based lubricant with glycerin (such as KY Jelly): These can dry up quickly, be sticky, and possibly lead to yeast infections, or irritate the vagina and be uncomfortable to women with vaginal sensitivities. However, these are the most commonly sold lubricants in pharmacies.
    - Water-based lubricant without glycerin: These can also be sticky and dry up quickly, but they are a healthy choice – they won't cause yeast infections or irritation. However, these might be more difficult to find – see our list of resources for places where you can find a large selection of lubricants.
    - Silicone-based lubricant: These are not sticky and are more long-lasting than water-based, though they're harder

to wash off and more expensive. These are also harder to find.

- If your water-based lubricant dries up, it's generally less messy to add some water to revitalize it, since adding more lubricant will make things more sticky.

- Too much of a good thing? Be careful not to overdo it in the lubrication department or you may find your sensations dulled.

- For women experiencing vaginal dryness, you can use a vaginal moisturizer (a lubricant bead that is inserted into the vagina prior to sex and can last for 24–48 hours) so that there is no need for an additional lubricant during sex.

- If you're trying to get pregnant, be aware that most commercial lubricants, as well as saliva, can kill sperm. If you want to use lubrication during this time, there is now a special conception-friendly lubricant on the market called Pre-Seed.

Do not buy a lubricant that contains lidocaine or benzocaine, as these ingredients numb the body to reduce discomfort. If you are feeling pain with intercourse, remember that pain is the body's signal telling you there is a problem, so go see a doctor!

Female Orgasm

Enjoying sex is an important part of your marriage, but it is equally important to realize that the presence or absence of orgasm does not always define great sex. Sex can be deep, meaningful, and connecting without an orgasm, and at times sex can be a not particularly satisfying or even a negative experience even with an orgasm. Be aware that current studies estimate that approximately 70 percent of all women who are sexually active are unable to experience an orgasm in the context of vaginal intercourse. Especially among women, the experience of orgasm isn't automatic or necessarily triggered by the same actions for every woman, so it can take a bit of exploring to find what works for you. Sexual exploration can be a fun process and something that deepens your knowledge of yourselves and your relationship as a couple.

The following paragraphs will help you learn about your body, and enhance the possibility of making orgasm a more comfortable part of your sex life.

Initially, take a look at illustration 1, showing female anatomy, and try touching the different labeled parts on yourself. See if any of them feel nice to the touch. You can also try – either by yourself or with your husband – touching yourself in different ways (i.e., stroking, gentle touch, massaging) to find the touch that feels most arousing to you. This may take some time and it also might be something that changes with time. Though the clitoris is the most sensitive part of the vulva, not every woman enjoys direct clitoral stimulation, and for some women indirect stimulation feels better. When preparing for this self-exploration, make sure that you're in a relaxed setting, whether it's your bed or in the bath (some women actually use the running water in a bath to bring themselves to orgasm), and give yourself/yourselves plenty of time to explore.

Just as in intercourse, touching your vagina when it isn't wet might feel uncomfortable, so you may want to use some lubricant (for more on lubricants see pages 37–39) or just apply some saliva before beginning. Also, you don't need to limit your explorations to your vagina alone – if your husband is with you, you may want to ask him to try stroking other parts of your body while you touch your vagina. You may find that this extra care and attention is all that you need to help you experience an orgasm.

If these suggestions don't help, or if you're already able to experience an orgasm on your own and are looking to experience it as part of intercourse, see pages 68–69.

We were wondering...

No Female Orgasm with Husband

SHE ASKS: While I've been able to experience an orgasm on my own, I find that I'm just not able to experience an orgasm when my husband is around (either during or apart from intercourse). Is there anything I can do to make things better?

At the beginning of marriage, everything is new, and learning to feel comfortable sexually in your husband's presence can take some time. In order to let go and have an orgasm, you need to be relaxed and comfortable in the situation. It may pay to do some emotional self-examination and ask yourself whether you can identify anything that's holding you back when your husband is around. If the situation doesn't improve with time, speak to a therapist.

Chapter 3

Alternate Intimacies

There may be times in your lives when having sexual intercourse is not ideal, for medical reasons or otherwise. While it may seem obvious to you that intercourse is not the sum total of your physical relationship, it is important to restate that point here. Hand-holding, hugs, kisses, and casual physical contact are all part of the way you express affection to one another, and these basic forms of intimacy should not be put on hold, even as you negotiate the time period that lies ahead.

In terms of more intense sexual activity, there is a wide range of sexual intimacies that you can enjoy as a couple. It is important to remember that vaginal intercourse is not the only type of sexual contact that exists, and while it may be your usual form of sexual contact, at certain times in the course of your marriage another form of sexual intimacy may be more comfortable. We will discuss a few basic options, though what follows is by no means exhaustive.

Though this guide has been prefaced with the caveat that it is not meant to serve as a halachic resource, this point deserves to be reiterated here. We have chosen to include below a wide range of sexual activities. However, some of the actions below may not be sanctioned by your individual *posek*.

Oral Stimulation

One thing you may want to try is oral sex. Since during oral sex, one partner uses the lips and tongue to bring the other partner sexual pleasure, personal hygiene is particularly important. Some people enjoy incorporating a bath or shower into their foreplay. Not everyone feels comfortable with oral sex, so it's important that you make sure you're both on the same page before giving this a try. Also note that oral sex does not need to culminate in orgasm; it can serve as foreplay leading into sexual intercourse.

When giving your wife oral sex, as with vaginal sex, engage in foreplay before beginning. If she's feeling self-conscious, it might help her feel more confident if you start while she's still wearing underpants. During oral sex you can use your tongue and lips on the various parts of her vulva. As with all sexual touch, this should start out gently and include communication about what does or does not feel good, as some parts of the vulva might be more sensitive than others and require a particular type of caress. Once you and your wife find the parts of the vagina that are most responsive to oral sex, you can experiment with different type of touches, such as licks, kisses, and nibbles, and different paces. She can also move her hips or caress her body while you are giving her oral sex, to enhance her pleasure.

In terms of giving your husband oral sex, you may want to start by using your tongue to lick your husband's penis. You can try licking it like a lollypop or moving it in and out of your mouth, mimicking a thrusting motion. Only take as much of the penis into your mouth as feels comfortable for you – trying to take too much of the penis in your mouth can cause a gag reflex for some people. As with your husband giving you oral sex, experiment with different types of licks and kisses and with different paces.

Oral sex is something that a husband and wife can give to each other separately or simultaneously. If you've never done this before, you may want to start by each trying to give each other oral sex independently, so that you can focus on being the giver or the receiver. Once you feel comfortable with it and if you're interested, you can try giving each other oral sex simultaneously, though not every couple will be able to configure their bodies for this (especially if one of you is significantly taller than the other). While some may enjoy this position, others may prefer to perform oral sex on each spouse individually, so as to fully enjoy both giving and receiving pleasure.

Manual Stimulation

Another option is to manually stimulate each other either with or without it culminating in orgasm. If you've never tried this before, it may be helpful to first watch your spouse touching him- or herself, so that you have a sense of the type and location of the caresses that your partner most enjoys. Feel free to use what you have seen your spouse doing, as well as to experiment with other types of touches. It is important that you both be open to each other's feedback as some types of stimulation may be uncomfortable. Figuring out how to manually pleasure your spouse is a learning process and may take some time, just as it took time to figure out how to have intercourse. You may want to also experiment with having your spouse stimulate his or her sexual organs while you touch other parts of his or her body, or stimulate yourselves in each other's presence.

You may find that you just enjoy watching your spouse's sexual pleasure, or you may want to join your spouse and experience the arousal and orgasm together. While there are many possibilities for such stimulation, if you're missing the mutuality of intercourse, you can try rubbing against each other to mimic the feelings of intercourse, or combine rubbing against each other with manual stimulation.

The key is to be open with yourselves and with each other, and to explore and find what feels good to both of you. While you may not have greeted a doctor's orders or your inability to engage in vaginal intercourse with joy, with open communication and a willingness to experiment, you may just find that a ban on intercourse allows you to learn new things together and find new avenues of sexual pleasure.

We were wondering...

BUYING SEXUAL ITEMS

THEY ASK: We are a very observant couple and live in a large religious community. Is there a discreet place where we can buy a vibrator or something else to enhance our sexual pleasure?

You can buy a range of sexual items discreetly online; however, not all websites that sell sexual items are trustworthy. For a few reputable websites, see our list of resources at the end of the manual.

Chapter 4

Time as a Factor in Your Intimate Lives

As observant Jews, you already know that much of your lives revolve around issues of time – when to say *Kriyat Shema*, when to start Shabbos, when to celebrate a *bar* or *bat mitzvah*. As you begin your lives as sexual partners, time will also play a key role in your expectations and behaviors. In this section, you will gain an awareness of this central factor and read about suggested ways to ease transitions and enhance your comfort level.

The moments when you stand together under the *chuppah* mark one of the most significant changes in your lives. Your becoming a married couple now allows you the opportunity to have a physical relationship with each other, including the intense, complex, and hopefully enjoyable experience of sexual intercourse. As we have discussed earlier, this transition can bring with it some feelings of anxiety and uncertainty. The time before the wedding and the time afterward represent two vastly different periods of your lives, and as you build your relationship together, other sexually related transitions await you.

Living with *Niddah*

One of your first transitions to consider will be the rhythm of *taharas hamishpachah*. Other than times of pregnancy and nursing, most religious couples will face the challenge of physically separating and then, about two weeks later, reconnecting every month. Adjusting to this pattern will take some time, patience, and goodwill, but it is well worth the effort. Adding to this challenge is the fact that you may have learned with different teachers and received different messages regarding

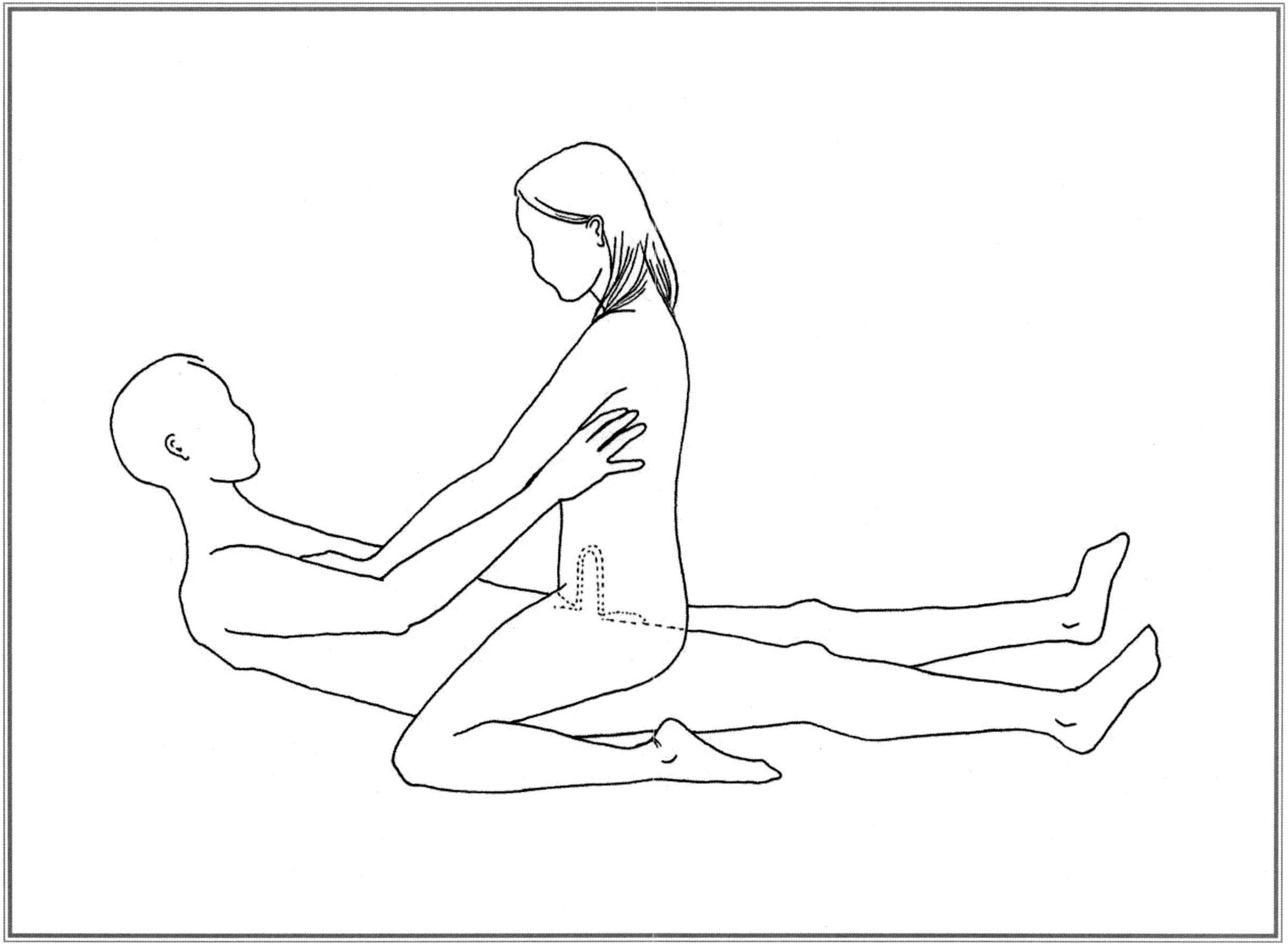

ILLUSTRATION 4: *Woman-on-top position*

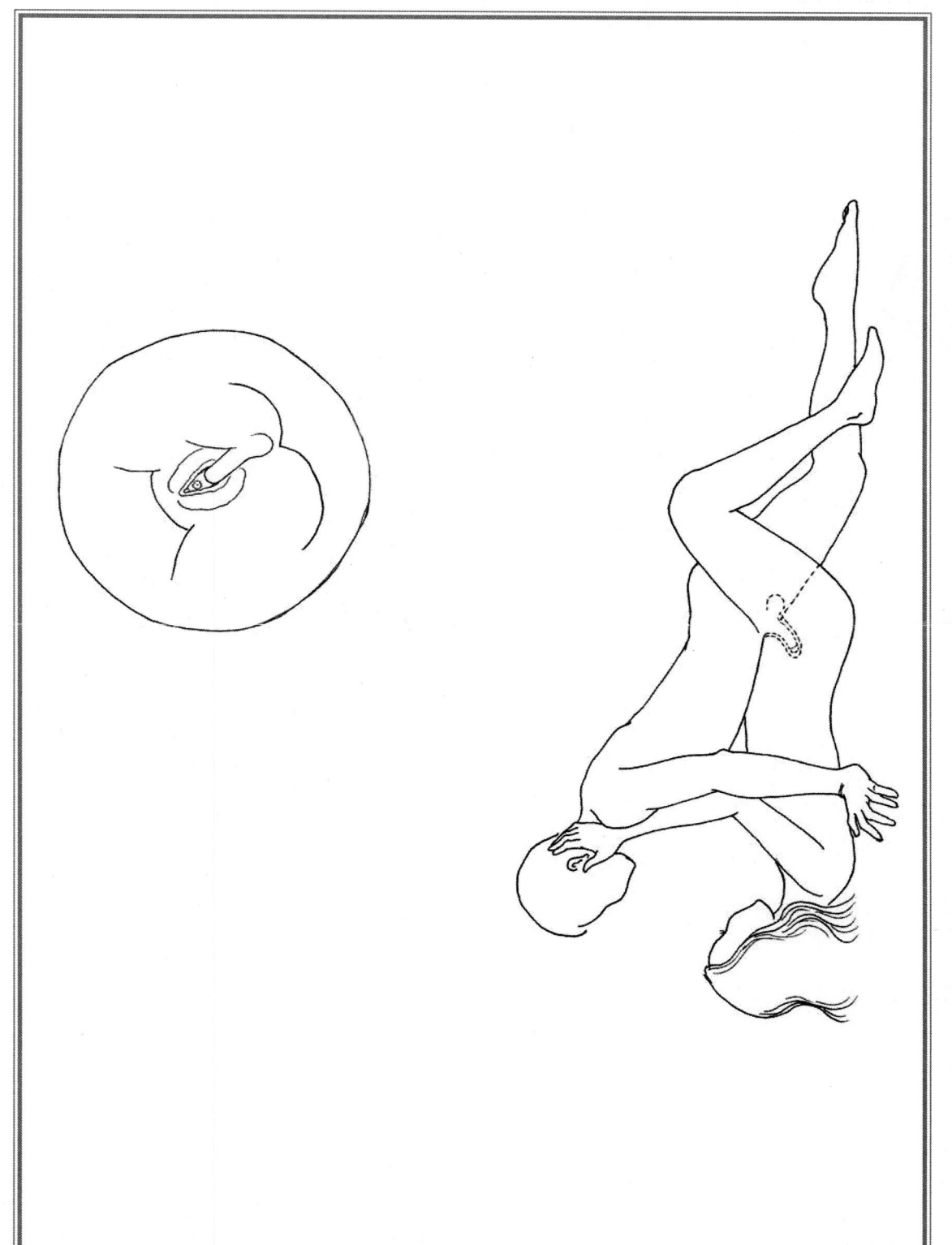

ILLUSTRATION 3: *Missionary position, with penetration close-up*

ILLUSTRATION 1: *Female vagina*

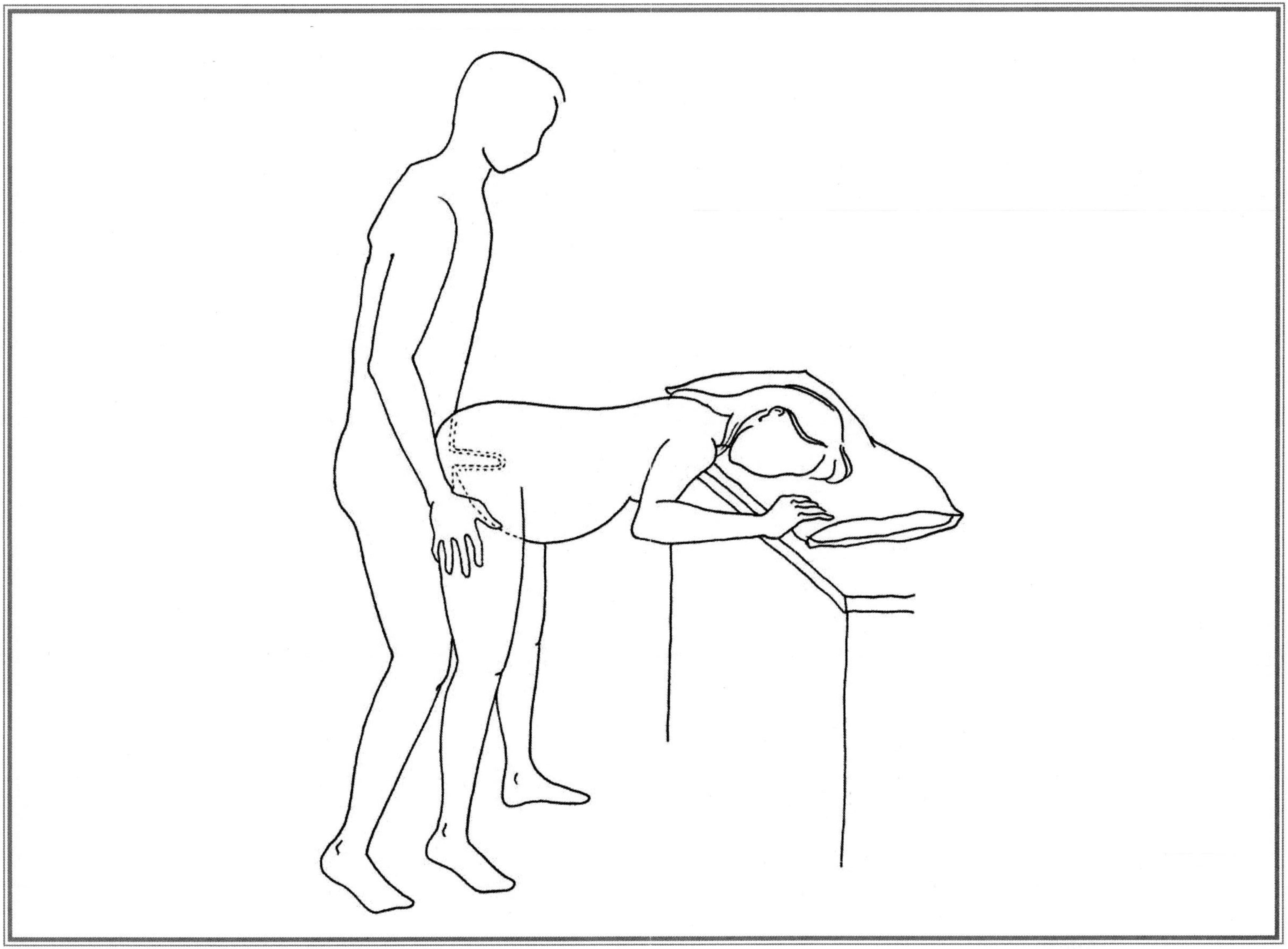

ILLUSTRATION 5: ***Rear-entry position (vaginal penetration)***

both *halachah* and *hashkafah*. Reaching a place comfortable for both of you will likely require open discussion and possibly consultation with a halachic authority.

How you view the time when you cannot touch goes a long way toward making these days easier on both of you. This is a shared *mitzvah* and shared experience, not just hers, and requires that you both invest a bit more in your non-physical relationship. During these two weeks, make a greater effort to be sensitive to each other, to be considerate and patient. Find time to spend with each other – learn something together, go for a walk, buy pizza, play a game. If refraining from touching causes stress to either of you, learn to gently share these feelings and to listen with understanding.

As *mikveh* night approaches, talk with each other about how to make those hours as pleasant and pleasurable as possible. For most women, getting accustomed to the *mikveh* experience takes some time. Learning the practical aspects of how and where to prepare, dealing with the discomfort of being naked in front of a *mikveh* attendant, and the possible anxiety of resuming sexual contact all require mutual understanding and time to adjust. Because *mikveh* is her *mitzvah*, he needs to be guided by whatever will make her life easier; doing the dishes while she gets ready and showering before she comes home from the *mikveh* are good ways to start.

Resuming your sex life after *mikveh* can be awkward; this is entirely to be expected. To ease back into this aspect of their lives, some couples make the evening into a special experience before they enter their bedroom, sharing a candlelit meal in their home, or engaging in another special activity together. When she returns from the *mikveh*, a gentle kiss, hug, or caress is a good way for each of you to say "welcome back." If starting foreplay then feels right to both of you, then go for it. If either of you needs more time to reconnect, explain your feelings and perhaps spend a while just holding hands, simply to get used to being physical again.

If returning to an active sex life after *mikveh* is truly fearful for either of you, that's the time to seek some help. See page 60 for guidelines about finding the right health professional.

Pregnancy

Other periods of time that will hopefully be part of your lives are the nine months of pregnancy, the time after delivery until *tevilah*, and the resumption of physical contact. Pregnancy allows for a break from the on/off schedule of *taharas hamishpachah*, and the extended time together can be enjoyable for both of you, but you may need to consider some other factors. A woman's hormonal and physical changes may have an impact on her sexual feelings. Women respond in various ways to being pregnant – and often the same woman will react differently in each pregnancy and in each trimester. Some women become more sexually desirous, some less, and others find that their level of desire remains the same. Whatever her response may be, it is important that he understand that she is not rejecting him; rather, the normal physiological and emotional effects of pregnancy can cause her nausea, exhaustion, and doubts about her physical attractiveness. For her part, she should be aware that most husbands do not see their wives as less attractive because of this normal change in the contours of their wives' bodies.

Sex can continue regularly throughout an uncomplicated pregnancy, unless your healthcare provider advises you otherwise. Sometimes husbands worry that sex might hurt the baby; this fear is totally ungrounded. If your usual sexual position is her on the bottom and him on top, you will probably need to change this as her stomach projects more during the developing pregnancy. One option commonly used by pregnant women is the female-on-top position (see page 69).

Another possible position to use during pregnancy is the rear-entry position. Achieving penetration in the rear-entry position can take some work on positioning – take a look at illustration 5 as you read the following. The woman's hips and shoulders need to be correctly aligned in order for this to work. One way to try this might be with the wife standing next to the bed and leaning forward on it with her buttocks raised up and with the husband standing behind her and penetrating. Depending on each of your heights, she might need to adjust the angle of her hips to bring her vaginal opening and his penis to the same level, or one of you may want to stand on a box (be sure to choose something stable) or phone book. She will also need to reach between her legs to guide his penis into her vagina in this position.

As an alternate way of using this position, the woman can be on her hands and knees in bed, with the man on his knees in back of her, his hips against her buttocks. Here too, she will need to guide his penis into her vagina.

We were wondering...

Sex during Pregnancy

HE ASKS: My wife is pregnant and has just begun to really show. I've heard that rear-entry is the best sexual position to use during pregnancy and the most comfortable for her (and our developing baby). However, we've tried this position a few times and it just hasn't felt comfortable for my wife. What should we do?

The best position to use during pregnancy is the one that is most comfortable for both of you. While the rear-entry position can definitely be a good idea during pregnancy, this position doesn't work for all women. For some, the deeper penetration that this position provides might be uncomfortable. And for others, it may be more difficult to reach orgasm in this position since the clitoris may not be stimulated. If the rear-entry position just isn't working for you,

you may want to try the woman-on-top position, which can also be comfortable to use during pregnancy (see illustration 4 and page 69 for more on this). Or you may want to try manually stimulating the clitoris while using the rear-entry position, to help your wife reach orgasm in this position (you may have to experiment with how to position your hands to make this work).

Postpartum

Many couples find that the period from delivery to *tevilah* requires a reworking of their relationship. Particularly for first-time parents, this new person in your lives will demand your time, energy, and patience, with regular sleep hours becoming just a memory. Sex may not be the first thing on either of your minds, but not hugging or caressing is often felt as particularly difficult. This can be especially challenging for her as she takes time to recover physically, to learn the skills of childcare, including nursing (if she is doing so), and to gradually resume her day-to-day functioning.

These weeks and months necessitate added mutual sensitivity and understanding. It is important that you see each other as full partners in this next stage of your lives and that you are prepared to offer an extra measure of emotional support. While it may seem an impossible fantasy at times, children eventually do sleep through the night and your lives will resume a sense of normalcy.

Your return to physical intimacy is marked by her first *tevilah*, anywhere from six weeks to three months after uncomplicated childbirth. Yet, though you are now permitted to be sexual, you may not quite feel up to resuming an active sex life. Some of the adjustment tasks of parenting may still be new and exhausting, leaving you with little energy for active sexual contact. Take your time; gradually get used to each other again, and consider alternate intimacies (see pages 42–44) if you don't feel ready for intercourse. Be open about your feelings and start at a pace comfortable for both of you. If the timing of your sex life before the birth of your baby had been primarily spontaneous, consider taking a more active role in planning opportunities to be together. This tends to reduce stress levels and provide a basis for ongoing physical intimacy.

Reconnecting sexually may be more difficult for her, particularly if she is nursing. There are now two people wishing intimate physical contact with her, which may cause unexpected and confusing feelings. The hormonal effects of nursing on a woman's body can also reduce sexual desire and cause vaginal dryness. In addition, the aftereffects of childbirth itself can lead to vaginal pain during intercourse, which may require a medical examination. In any of these situations, honest communication is the best place to start. All of this may be frightening, and you will need each other's understanding and support.

We were wondering...

POSTPARTUM SEX

THEY ASK: We had our first baby several months ago and everything in our lives has changed since then, including our sexual relationship. As a new father I find that I'm often too tired to even think about sex, and when I do, the desire surfaces as more of a physiological need than a desire for intimacy. As a new mother, I am overwhelmed by exhaustion at the end of the day and just want to catch a few hours of sleep before the baby wakes up again. In addition, my body also feels worn out from the childbirth experience and from the intensive demands of breastfeeding... And even those times when we do end up having sex, I find that I'm not able to enjoy it as much as I did before our baby was born. Are we normal? And is there a way to salvage our sexual relationship during this stage in our lives?

> *THEY ASK: We had our first baby several months ago and have been challenged by the different ways that each of us has responded to that experience. As the woman, I have been feeling more of a desire for closeness and reassurance — but less so for sex. As the man, I have been feeling an increased desire for intimacy; my wife spends so much time caring for the baby that I need some reassurance that I'm still loved. How can we work this out?*

It is important to emphasize that you're certainly not alone in your feelings and experience. One or both of you may feel less interested in sex at this time — in general you have less time and energy to devote to intimacy during this phase. The postpartum period is often characterized by the challenge of balancing your new family life with your relationship as a couple, and there are no easy solutions. Sexual relationships change over the course of your marriage and this is one of those times. Eventually, you will adjust to the baby and find a new pattern for your sexual relationship. In the interim, don't give up on physical contact altogether, as hugging and cuddling at the end of a long day can reassure you both that you still love each other.

One issue that is important to stress is that if the woman is feeling pain during intercourse, it should be checked out with a doctor until the issue is fully resolved. Pain should not be ignored even in the spirit of compromise; until the pain is resolved, explore alternate forms of intimacy (see pages 42–44).

Baby Interrupting Lovemaking

> *THEY ASK: We really love our baby, but sometimes when we want to be intimate, he seems to know and starts to cry in the middle. After one of us returns from calming him down, getting started again rarely seems to work.*

Welcome to the world of parenting and discovering things no one told you. While your child will eventually sleep through the night, until that time, the baby waking and interrupting you in the midst of intimate moments can be very unsettling. When this happens, usually one of you will tend to your infant, while the other waits, often with diminishing patience and sexual desire. While there is no foolproof solution, two things may help. First, this would be the right time to use your sense of humor to ease the tension and at least feel relaxed with each other. Second, try getting up together to deal with the childcare tasks, allowing you to maintain some level of connection and preventing either of you from feeling left alone in your bedroom. Some ongoing gentle touch at this time can go a long way toward maintaining the sexual mood.

Chapter 5

When Your Sex Life Isn't Working

Despite your good health and goodwill, either or both of you may encounter situations that cannot be fixed through any of the suggestions we have offered in previous sections. These can happen to any of us, but fortunately, most can be helped by a trained and certified sexual health professional. What follows is a brief description of some of these problems, and then some guidelines as to how to find the right source of help. *In almost all of these situations, your first stop should be your medical doctor.*

It is important to note that while some of these conditions may limit sexual activity, they will not prevent you from enjoying alternate options for physical intimacy, as we have described earlier. Equally crucial will be the understanding and support that you show each other during this sensitive time.

Men's Concerns

ERECTILE DYSFUNCTION (ED)

No sexual response happens every time you want it to; sometimes you may be too tired or too focused on things that worry you. If he usually is able to have an erection, but sometimes it doesn't work, he's normal. If he cannot have an erection most of the time you are sexually active, speak to a sexual health professional. This condition is called Erectile Dysfunction and can be caused by physical or emotional factors, or a combination of both. A number of treatment options are currently available, including prescription medications such as Viagra, Cialis, and Levitra. These medications enhance his body's ability to send blood to the penis, making it easier for him to have an erection when he is aroused. Just a word of caution: these medications must be prescribed by a physician and taken under his or her care. Do not borrow some pills from your brother-in-law, do not order them online, and do not be fooled by "natural" remedies.

RAPID OR PREMATURE EJACULATION (PE)

When sexually active with their partners, some men may regularly ejaculate before penetration, while others may ejaculate within a minute or less after thrusting begins. This condition is called premature or rapid ejaculation and is quite common. If this occurs primarily after a prolonged time without sexual contact, such as on *mikveh* night or after a period of illness, it is entirely normal and is not a cause for concern. Additionally, some men will be able to have a second erection soon after they ejaculate and last longer the second time. If the PE is frequent and interferes with your sexual pleasure as a couple, it is time to get some help. Treatment is either through exercises the two of you do at home or through taking medication. For further information see pages 72–74.

MALE ORGASMIC DISORDER (MOD)

This condition occurs when a man can achieve erection and engage in sexual intercourse, but cannot reach orgasm/ejaculation no matter how long a time the thrusting continues. MOD prevents conception and may cause physical discomfort for both husband and wife. At this point, the only treatment option is through behavioral sex therapy techniques, with additional therapy sessions to deal with possible emotional issues. If the condition persists, the couple should consult with a fertility clinic.

Women's Concerns

VAGINISMUS

If you experience tightness and/or pain around the vaginal opening, or find it difficult or impossible to allow penetration, despite your desire to do so, you may have vaginismus. This condition is more common among women new to sexual intercourse but may also appear after childbirth or be related to other medical or emotional causes. Vaginismus is often the cause of unconsummated marriages (marriages in which intercourse has not yet taken place). A medical examination is the first stop, with treatment done either by your doctor or a physical therapist trained to deal with women's sexual issues. This is a treatable condition, so don't assume you can never enjoy sexual intercourse.

Painful Intercourse

Estimates are that at some point in their lives most women will experience painful intercourse, albeit for a brief period of time. The pain may range from mildly uncomfortable to absolutely intolerable, and may be caused by a wide variety of factors, physical and emotional. If solutions such as added lubrication or modifying/changing a sexual position do not help, immediately stop whatever activity is causing the pain. Medical examination is the next step and should happen as soon as possible. The good news is that relief is available in almost all cases; do not hesitate to follow through on treatment recommendations.

Concerns for Either Men or Women

Aversion and/or Lack of Interest

Feeling strange and uncomfortable during your first few sexual experiences is only to be expected. Touching someone else's body or having your body touched, especially in the most private and intimate places, does not come easily to everyone. There may be some, however, who have little or no desire for physical touch or cannot tolerate any kind of sexual experience. There are many potential causes for this condition and each requires its own kind of therapy, some of which may be lengthy. Getting you both to a healthier place will require your best efforts at mutual support and understanding during the course of therapy.

MEDICAL CONDITIONS AND MEDICATIONS

Some medical conditions not directly related to the sexual organs may have an impact on sexual desire and performance. Sometimes the effect is related to a specific medical situation, such as diabetes or kidney dysfunction requiring renal dialysis. In other situations, emotional factors may play the central role, such as recovering heart attack patients fearful of resuming sexual activity. In addition, medications may have a negative sexual influence, such as some medications used to treat depression or high blood pressure, or some types of birth control pills. In many of these instances, your doctor can suggest an alternate treatment or medication, add a medication, or offer a referral to a sex therapist to restore the potential for sexual satisfaction.

CHILDHOOD SEXUAL ABUSE

Victims of childhood sexual abuse exist in every society, although we may try to pretend it only happens to a mythical "*them.*" Abuse includes more than just instances of an adult forcing intercourse on a child. Any inappropriate sexual touch or speech or exposure to pornographic material may cause traumatic damage with the potential to impact negatively on sexual expectations and responses later in life. At times, these memories are so painful that we cannot consciously recall them, but they may cause behavioral or emotional symptoms. Although a certain percentage of survivors are not affected by prior abuse, some of these victims may experience difficulties. Some examples are unwillingness to be touched physically, fear of giving or receiving any sexual contact, recurring nightmares with sexual themes, or unexplained crying episodes. If either of you suspects you may have suffered sexual abuse, it is imperative that you seek help as soon as possible.

Negative Body Image

Regrettably, we live in a time when expectations of physical appearance have taken on damaging proportions. We have been told countless times that unless we look like Hollywood stars or Olympic athletes, there is something wrong with us. Such perceptions may influence our comfort level with our own bodies and our expectations of how others (for example, a husband or wife) should look. We may say *sheker hachen v'hevel hayofi*, but we often don't believe it. Compounding the problem is a tendency that many of us have to be overly critical of how our bodies appear; we only see the negative and assume that is what others see as well. Any such feelings can adversely affect your comfort level with yourself or your partner, both physically and emotionally. This is a difficult and often painful issue to discuss, especially if it relates to your perception of your spouse's body. In this case, whoever is bothered by this should first seek individual counseling before discussing the matter with his or her spouse.

Homosexuality

The topic of homosexuality is a highly charged one within the religious community and this book is not the place for a full discussion. However, it is important to note that same-sex attraction seems to affect a small percentage of all populations and thus may be a cause for sexual incompatibility in a marriage; a lack of sexual desire and arousal may be due to an inability to have sexual feelings about someone of the opposite sex. This is not always an automatic reason to end a marriage, but it clearly indicates an immediate need to get some help. One important note: homosexual content in dreams or fantasies is not necessarily an indication of homosexual desire or orientation.

Pornography

We are using the term *pornography* here although there is no clear definition for this term and much still needs to be learned about this topic.

The internet's providing access to almost endless sources of sexually explicit material has become increasingly worrisome to the religious community. While acknowledging the validity of this concern, it is important to point out that: (1) men and women may view pornography very differently, and this in itself may be a source of conflict that needs to be addressed, and (2) viewing pornography should not automatically be defined as an addictive behavior. Beyond the complex problems associated with viewing pornography, it can also cause a serious breach of trust within a marriage. If you are dealing with this challenge in your relationship, start off by discussing the topic together, as uncomfortable as this may be, and don't hesitate to turn to professionals for help if the problem persists. Pornography may not be related to sexual satisfaction in your marriage, so don't assume that all is lost.

We were wondering...

SPOUSE PRESSURING ME

SHE ASKS: We've only been married for three months, and almost since day one my husband has been forcing me into sexual acts and positions that I feel uncomfortable with. I've tried saying no, but he often won't take no for an answer. What should I do?

The right to say no to any given sexual request is basic to the trust required for a successful marriage, whether you've been together for a day, a week, or fifty years. If your husband is unable to respect your "no" (sexual or otherwise) then it's time to get help from a mental health professional as soon as possible. If your husband tries to prevent you from speaking to a therapist, call an abuse hotline immediately.

Working with a Sex Therapist

THEY ASK: We've been married for nearly a year and have been experiencing some problems in our sex life, so we've decided to see a sex therapist. However, it's not the type of professional we can ask anyone to recommend, so we're trying to find someone online. Is there anything we should be aware of before we start seeing him or her?

It's great that you're taking control of the situation by asking for help. Though it may be initially uncomfortable, your rabbi may be able to recommend a sex therapist with whom he has worked in the past and who is sensitive to the needs of an Orthodox couple. Indeed, you may end up finding a better therapist this way than by simply looking online. Your medical doctor might also be a good person to ask for a referral to a sex therapist. Either way, there are a few things that can be helpful to know before seeing a sex therapist:

- A sex therapist will ask you intimate questions about your sex life in order to help you. However, unless the sex therapist is also a medical doctor (which is rare) or a physical therapist or a nurse, you should never be asked to remove your clothing. If this does happen, you should leave.

- Being open and honest in the therapist's office is important. Even though some of the questions asked may be personal, honesty is the best way to bring you closer to solving your problem.

- Sex therapists will often meet with each member of the couple separately after meeting with them together. This will help the therapist understand each person's individual issues.

- Before sex therapy can start, any underlying medical problems need to be addressed. After discussing with you the reason for the visit, the sex therapist will be able to give you specific instructions about the type of medical evaluation you need to have carried out by an appropriate medical professional.

- The therapist may give you "homework" to practice at home. The homework may consist of "sensate focus exercises," which may be fun to try even if you don't have a problem but just want to learn more about your own or your spouse's body.

- Working with a therapist who does not share your religious values may require you to take the time to explain these fundamental aspects of your lives. If it is comfortable for you, your rabbi can also be helpful in these situations, and most therapists would be happy to consult with him.

Part 2

Beyond the Basics: Tips and Advice

This section contains practical advice about a range of sexual issues, and is structured like the *"We were wondering…"* sections in part 1 of this book. We hope that the more personal nature of the questions and answers in this section can help normalize your own concerns as well as give you practical tips and advice for dealing with them.

The first chapter of this section is oriented specifically toward women and women's concerns, the second specifically toward men and men's concerns, and the third to concerns that both husband and wife may share. We recommend that you read this entire section and not just issues addressed to your gender; reading the section on "She Asks" can help you as a husband understand some of your wife's concerns, and reading the section on "He Asks" can help you as a wife understand some of your husband's concerns. Cross-references to part 1 will also be provided in order to make sure you have all the information readily accessible.

Chapter 6

She Asks

Preparing Your Body for the First Sexual Experience

> SHE ASKS: *I'm really nervous about our first sexual experience and was hoping that there was something I could do in advance to prepare my body. Any suggestions?*

Remember that you're marrying someone with whom you want to share your life and you've probably been looking forward to this experience for a long time. Getting overly worked up about your first sexual experience risks becoming a self-fulfilling prophecy.

One piece of advice that may bring you to the first sexual experience feeling more relaxed and ready is taking some time to practice inserting a tampon while you are lying down on your back. Even if you've used tampons for years, you've most likely inserted them while either standing or sitting on the toilet. Inserting a tampon while lying down can feel different and will help to prepare you for the experience of penetration.

Find a time when you won't be disturbed and can be assured of having some privacy in your own room. While lying down on your back, insert some lubricant (see pages 37-39) into your vagina or rub some on the tampon and then insert the tampon. Using a tampon with a plastic applicator may be easier. You can also try buying a box that contains tampons of different sizes so that you can begin by inserting the smallest and work your way up to the largest. This can give you some sense of what to expect during penetration and allow you to approach your wedding night feeling more at ease and excited. This can also be a time to get to know your own body so that you'll be better prepared to guide your husband in pleasuring you.

First Sexual Experience – Painful or Not?

SHE ASKS: I've heard that the first sexual experience can be painful for women – is this true? Is there anything I can do to make my first sexual experience more comfortable?

There is a certain amount of pressure you will probably feel during the first penetration due to the stretching of the hymen. The hymen is a membrane located close to the vaginal entrance (without any biological function that anybody is aware of). The exact structure and even location of the hymen varies greatly from woman to woman. For most women the hymen is perforated before puberty to allow for menstrual blood to exit the body. People often speak of feeling "pressure" as opposed to "pain" when the hymen stretches or tears – though, in your first sexual experience, when you've never before felt the sensation of having a penis inside your vagina, how can you really know the difference? You should probably be prepared to feel some discomfort, even if you are relaxed and aroused.

Though it is normal to feel some pain in one's first sexual experience, getting overly worked up in anticipation will only turn into a self-fulfilling prophecy. Here's why: every woman has a series of muscles surrounding her vagina (called pubococcygeus or PC muscles), and when she feels stress or anxiety those muscles may become tense and she physically may not be able to let her husband's penis enter. Being relaxed and aroused ensures that the PC muscles will also relax, making it easier for your husband to penetrate. Often a painful or failed attempt at penetration will only make subsequent attempts more difficult (as the PC muscles may tighten in anticipation of a repeat performance), so don't try it until you really feel ready. And remember, you're not in a hurry. Take your time and try to begin discovering what makes each of you feel good; this is a learning process and it will get better with time...

In the initial sexual experiences, using a lubricant can also make things more comfortable. For more on lubrication, see pages 37–39.

No Female Orgasm

> SHE ASKS: *We've been married for a few months and I feel like we've tried everything but I still haven't had an orgasm – my husband has tried touching my vagina and clitoris but nothing seems to work, and we're just about ready to give up. Is there anything else we can try?*

Firstly, don't be alarmed and don't give up – just about all women are eventually able to have an orgasm. Enjoying sex is an important part of your marriage, so don't lose hope after only a couple of months of effort.

We'll list two suggestions below, which you should feel free to try in the order that seems most comfortable for you. Given that sex is still new for you, the suggestions below may seem uncomfortable or embarrassing for you to try right away. Try talking to your husband about whether you might feel comfortable exploring these options together (see pages 23–25 for more on sexual communication and how to begin this type of conversation).

The first option is oral stimulation: sometimes the tongue and lips are able to provide a more subtle and sensitive touch than the hand and fingers and bring women to orgasm when manual stimulation cannot. For more about how your husband can give you oral sex, see pages 42–43.

Another option is a vibrator. Vibrators come in different shapes and sizes (some are primarily for external clitoral stimulation, and some, shaped like a penis, are designed primarily for penetration) with different types of mechanics (some are battery powered, some run on AC power and either need to be plugged into an outlet or are rechargeable). The basic idea is that a vibrator – unlike a hand or finger – provides continuous stimulation, which can give some women an orgasm when nothing else can. But don't underestimate the importance of relaxation and fantasy. Most women use a vibrator externally and are able to reach orgasm by placing the vibrator on the clitoral area. Like anything new, a vibrator may take some getting used to, before you find a way of using it that works for you. Once you have it figured out, you can also use a vibrator on yourself during intercourse, or teach your husband how to use it to enhance your pleasure either during or apart from intercourse. See the resources section for a list of websites where you can purchase a vibrator.

No Female Orgasm during Intercourse

> SHE ASKS: *We've been married for a couple of years now and though I'm generally able to reach orgasm through clitoral stimulation, I've never been able to have an orgasm during intercourse. I know the statistics – that something like 70 percent of women can't have an orgasm during intercourse – but I'd still like to try to make it happen. Do you have any suggestions that might help us?*

If you find that even after being able to experience an orgasm by yourself, you are still not able to do so during intercourse, here are a few questions you can ask yourself: Is enough foreplay taking place? (Keep in mind that many women need more foreplay before feeling aroused than men.) Are you feeling aroused and lubricated when intercourse begins? If not, this could be the reason why you're not reaching orgasm during intercourse, so try spending more time on foreplay before your husband attempts penetration.

If that doesn't seem to be the issue, you may want to ask yourself whether sex is happening too quickly for you – is your husband ejaculating soon after penetration? Or, is he able to maintain thrusting for a sustained period of time (the average is 4–5 minutes), but the thrusting just isn't doing anything for you? If your husband is a rapid ejaculator (see pages 55, 72–74), you may need to work on that first, before reading the suggestions that follow. If, however, your husband is able to maintain thrusting for a sustained period of time, you may want to try to increase the clitoral stimulation that you are getting during intercourse in order to help you reach orgasm.

To do so, positioning is important. The position most conducive to clitoral stimulation (without any extra effort on your part) is the man-on-top position (see illustration 3). Using this position, when your husband's penis is fully inside of you, his pubic bone should rub against your clitoris as he thrusts during intercourse, thus giving you the clitoral stimulation you need. You can also move your hips or legs, or position a pillow beneath your hips to adjust the angle so that your husband's pubic bone will stimulate your clitoris more directly while he is thrusting. This might take some figuring out. Having your husband's support is really important – open communication is essential to making this work!

Another suggestion would be to try an alternate sexual position, namely, the woman-on-top position (see illustration 4, as this position is not merely a reversal of the man-on-top position). In this position your husband is lying down on his back and you sit on top of him with your knees on the bed on either side of him. Just be aware that this position may be awkward for new couples who aren't yet fully comfortable being naked with each other, as the woman's entire body is exposed. The major advantage here is that both you and your husband will have your hands free, so that either he or you can manually (or with a vibrator) stimulate the clitoris or the labia during intercourse. If you are interested in more suggestions about reaching orgasm – either during or apart from intercourse – see pages 39–41.

Mikveh Night Difficulty – Turning Back On

> SHE ASKS: *We have worked hard to maintain a good sense of intimacy during the* niddah *times when we can't touch, but I am finding it difficult to have any sexual desire for my husband on* mikveh

> *night. Although I feel more positive after a few days, the switch from being not sexual to sexual every month is often very difficult.*

Because you are human and not a light switch, turning off and then turning on each month may not always feel natural. For many women this is a particularly difficult time, since the resumption of physical intimacy rests on the outcome of her *bedikos*, and anxiety about possible staining and the prolonging of the *niddah* period can easily reduce sexual desire. Allowing sufficient time after you are married to get used to this rhythm often helps, as does your husband's patience and understanding.

When you feel you may need something to augment the mood, we suggest that you start planning for *mikveh* night as soon as you start counting *shiv'ah neki'im*. At first, let yourself begin to think about the kind of intimate touch you have enjoyed in the past, then build gradually to imagining being with your husband, doing whatever gives you a good feeling. Sharing some of this with your husband on the day of *tevilah* may enhance the atmosphere for both of you.

On the physical side, the *bedikos* that you do for a week before *tevilah* may have a function beyond the needs of *taharas hamishpachah*. Perhaps this presents the opportunity for you to reconnect with yourself sexually, before you renew your physical intimacy with your husband. Touching your vaginal area, outside and inside, while thinking intimately of your husband, could ease the transition back to the comfort and enjoyment of a regular sex life. If doing *bedikos* seems like the wrong time for you to reconnect with your sexual feelings, make an effort to find other times during that week that feel more comfortable for you – perhaps bathing before you begin the *shiv'ah neki'im*, or using the time in the bath before you go to the *mikveh* to fantasize and touch yourself might work better.

Chapter 7

He Asks

Not Able to Get an Erection

> HE ASKS: *We've been married for a few days, and have not been able to consummate our marriage yet. The problem seems to be that I'm just not able to get an erection. I've never had this problem in the past and we're both really confused – is there something wrong with me?*

Don't worry – what you're experiencing happens to lots of other *chassanim*. The fact that you've been able to have an erection in the past is a good sign, and your inability to have an erection now is likely a result of the anxiety that you're feeling at this time. It's completely normal to be feeling uncertain about the first sexual experience – but the way your body works is that anxiety actually serves to make it more difficult for you to achieve an erection.

The first step in relaxing is to try to take the stress off of having sex right now, because, ironically, once you know you are not required to have intercourse, it may actually be easier for you to do so. Some ways to relax include just changing the scenery, going for a leisurely walk together, taking a bubble bath together if you both feel comfortable (you can always wear a bathing suit if you are not yet ready to bathe together without any clothes), sharing a little wine or champagne (a little bit of alcohol can help to relax you, though too much may have a negative effect on your sexual functioning), or just doing something different to take the focus off sex for a time and help you feel more at ease.

Once you are feeling relaxed and ready to try again, it's important to take your time with foreplay, and allow yourself to become aroused before attempting penetration again. For a definition and some suggestions regarding foreplay, you may want to look at the first part of this manual, or put the books aside and just use your imagination and see what feels best to both of you. If she is sufficiently comfortable, your wife may want to try manual or oral stimulation of your penis to help you reach an erection. If none of these suggestions are able to help, a sexual health professional may suggest the temporary use of medication. While not being able to have an erection can feel embarrassing, frightening, or confusing, it is something that most men experience at some point in their lives and that will likely resolve itself once you're feeling more relaxed.

Rapid Ejaculation

> HE ASKS: *We've been married for several months, and I always ejaculate either soon after penetration occurs or sometimes before we're even able to achieve penetration. When this happened our first time together, I figured that it would go away as we had more experience, but it's been a few months and I think we would both enjoy sex more if I could last longer. What can I do?*

Firstly, you should know that rapid ejaculation is something that many men experience occasionally over the course of their lives. However, for the sake of your relationship at this point, it's important to separate the issue of your rapid ejaculation from the issue of your being able to pleasure your wife, and deal with each of these on its own.

Pleasuring your wife does not have to be linked to sexual intercourse, and until you're able to maintain better ejaculatory control, you may want to focus on pleasuring your wife through vaginal stimulation before or after intercourse. See pages 42–44 for more discussion on female sexuality and ways to do this.

It's important to understand that rapid ejaculation can happen due to a variety of causes, so not everything written here will necessarily apply to you. Some people experience rapid ejaculation due to the newness of the situation. Being sexually intimate with your wife is something that you have been so eager for that your body just moves through the process quickly. If this category seems to describe you, then you may find that with time and just getting used to the sexual relationship, the problem goes away on its own. It may also help to try an alternate sexual position, such as the woman on top, in which some men feel that ejaculation can be delayed longer.

Alternatively, you may find that there are times when rapid ejaculation recurs, such as *mikveh* night, when you return from an extended trip, or other times when you have not engaged in sex for a prolonged period of time. Understanding this may make it easier for you and your wife to come up with a plan that takes this into account. For example, you may find that on *mikveh* night you experience rapid ejaculation the first time you have sex, but after waiting for a while you may be able to have sex again and this time be able to last longer. Or, you may decide that on *mikveh* night you will first pleasure your wife in ways that don't require intercourse.

Another type of rapid ejaculation can result from how you have approached sexuality in the past. If your main sexual experiences have been with masturbation, this may have been an activity that you attempted to do in the shortest amount of time. Since your body has become accustomed to responding quickly, it may take some time for it to be rewired to changing circumstances and to be able to slow down. Often, knowledge is power, and with a little more knowledge about the sexual response process, you may be able to overcome this problem. This new learning is best done with the help of a therapist who can guide you through a series of exercises.

Regardless of the causes of your rapid ejaculation, open communication with your wife is a good first step. As long as you are both silent, the problem can feel overwhelming, especially if you are trying to become more self-aware and to understand how your body works. At the end of the day, you may even find that working through this issue together as a new couple has deepened your relationship and brought you closer together.

Mikveh Night Exhaustion

> HE ASKS: *Sometimes I get nervous as* mikveh *night approaches, and I worry about whether I can meet my wife's expectations. I usually come home tired after a long day and sometimes upset about how the day has gone. Occasionally, I find that I'm just not in the mood when my wife returns from the* mikveh. *What can I do?*

One of the challenges with scheduling sex, such as *mikveh* night, is that your moods do not always match the calendar. While *mikveh* night should be a time of reconnection and even celebration, busy and sometimes stressful lives may diminish your desire for intimacy. Try to understand the challenges each of you faces in your daily lives, and be patient and understanding when your moods don't happen to fit the schedule.

If anticipation of *mikveh* night usually makes you feel anxious, you may want to consider some changes. Perhaps you can change your schedule on the day of *mikveh* night, coming home early enough to relax, get some rest, and take some time to disconnect from the day's demands. If the nights present a problem, discuss with each other the possibility of making use of morning time to return to your sex life. Getting up earlier together, when you are rested and the world is quieter, can become an especially intimate occasion for both of you and perhaps become a regular time for sexual activity.

Chapter 8

They Ask

Guilt from Prior Sexual Experiences

> THEY ASK: *We've been married for a few months and I'm still feeling challenged in the sexual realm. All of my past sexual experiences happened alone – in the context of masturbation – engendering worries about issur and major guilt. How do I make the mental switch to partnered sexuality?*

> THEY ASK: *Neither of us was able to live up to being strictly shomer negi'ah before our marriage. For both of us, sexuality was often experienced as a source of shame and guilt. How can we leave that baggage behind us as we begin our sexual relationship together?*

Issues of shame, guilt, and other painful emotions have the potential to limit anyone's capacity to experience sex as a positive element of their marital relationship. While this manual emphasizes the fulfilling and nurturing aspects of physical intimacy, for some, this may seem a difficult goal, especially in the beginning.

Keep in mind that many of your past experiences were probably the result of normal sexual curiosity; human beings aren't perfect. Life is a process and without our pasts, we would never have become who we are today. If you can view your previous sexual experiences in the context of your own personal process of growth and development, you can put your past in a positive framework, and be ready for the next step.

Marriage is a new beginning for both of you; it is a chance to build a positive and healthy sexual relationship that will last a lifetime. Take what you have learned from your past and use it to help you move forward into a more positive place. Talk with each other about the type of sexual connection that you want to create with each other, and work together to make that a reality.

While guilt can sometimes seem all-consuming and overwhelming, it's critical that you not lose sight of your spouse amidst these powerful emotions. Try discussing your feelings with each other, and listening with support and empathy. You might want to try learning together the Jewish sources that speak about sexual intimacy between husband and wife in positive terms. Being able to articulate and work through your feelings together as a couple can go a long way toward easing your feelings of past guilt and making the transition into a positive and uplifting sexual relationship. As with any transition, changing your mentality in this realm won't necessarily happen overnight, so be patient with yourselves and with each other.

However, if you find that these negative feelings are not going away or are getting worse, you should seek the help of a therapist specializing in this area, ideally in consultation with a rabbi.

Transitioning from No Touch to Full Intercourse

> THEY ASK: *We're getting married next week and have remained* shomer negi'ah *throughout our dating and engagement. In thinking about our wedding night, it seems like too much to jump from no physical contact at all to full intercourse and then back to no touch all in one night. How can we make this transition?*

The transition from no contact to sex and back again all in one night can be truly daunting. Many couples do not have intercourse on their wedding night, and if you both feel more comfortable taking things slowly, that's fine. Be sure to communicate with each other about how you feel and what you want.

If you decide to delay intercourse, you should discuss with your rabbi what will happen if your wife gets her period before penetration has occurred, and the halachic implications of partial penetration. Similarly, you should discuss with your doctor issues of setting the wedding date and the time of your next period in a manner that gives you enough time to consummate the marriage. If you are taking medication to help set your wedding date, discuss in detail with both your doctor and rabbi the possibility of having extra pills on hand in case it takes some time to consummate the marriage.

Difficulty with Penetration

> THEY ASK: *We've been married for a few days, but every time we attempt penetration, it feels like he's reaching a closed door and can't enter at all – is this how it's supposed to be? Could it be that his penis is just too big to fit inside my vagina? Are we normal?*

Many newly married couples need some time before they are able to have full sexual relations. Especially on the wedding night, and the week of *Sheva Brachos* that follows, both of you may be physically and emotionally exhausted. These feelings are important to discuss with each other, and you should not expect to necessarily consummate your marriage on the first night, even if both of you want to do so.

In terms of his feeling like he's reaching a closed door when attempting penetration, there are a few steps you can take to become more comfortable and make penetration possible. It's helpful for both of you to become aroused before attempting penetration again – this whole experience is new and it's important to be patient with yourselves. Take it slow, talk with each other, and enjoy yourselves in the process.

Before attempting penetration again, she may want to try to insert one or two fingers into her vagina or have him do so, so that she can experience what it is like to have something inside her vagina, and feel that there is enough room for his penis. This suggestion, however, is not for everyone; if you don't feel comfortable trying it, then don't.

Occasionally, however, the feeling you describe might signal a problem that requires professional help. If even superficial vaginal touch produces pain and/or if she is not able to tolerate having anything inserted into her vagina (be it a tampon, a finger, or a penis), seek help from a sexual health professional right away.

Not Ready for Intercourse

> THEY ASK: *We're in the middle of our* Sheva Brachos *and we are still having a hard time with intimacy. We both enjoyed our first hugs and kisses, but we just don't feel comfortable with attempting sexual intercourse yet. What should we do?*

At this point in your marriage, any physical contact may be a new experience, and your feelings of hesitation are normal. While you don't feel ready to consummate the marriage right now, the fact that you've both enjoyed your initial mutual touch is a good sign, and perhaps all you both need is to take things slowly and not feel pressured – sometimes once the pressure is removed, it's easier to feel desire. An important element to consider is that of romance: feeling like you must have sex as soon as possible is not the best recipe for putting either of you into a romantic mood. Sexuality is intimately connected with emotions and state of mind. So why not try creating a romantic atmosphere in the tiny bit of free time you have during *Sheva Brachos*, whether you go for a quiet walk, hold hands, or just cuddle on the couch.

Another important element is that you both feel sexually aroused and physically prepared for intercourse. The best way to do so is by making sure to engage in mutually enjoyable sexual activity and communicating about what feels most pleasurable before attempting intercourse. You can also read the section on foreplay (page 29) for more ideas and information.

Frequency of Sex

> THEY ASK: *We've been married for almost a year and still haven't figured out how often we should be having sex — is there a standard amount that we should be aiming for? And, should we decide in advance when to have relations, or is it better for it to be more spontaneous?*

This is perhaps one of the most asked questions, but really one that has no right or wrong answer. Figuring out a rhythm to your sexual life varies widely from couple to couple. One of the most challenging and rewarding aspects to the beginning of marriage is navigating this uncharted territory and figuring out what works for you both. Keep in mind that intimacy includes a wide range of experiences beyond intercourse, and that your individual needs for intimacy might not always include intercourse (see the section on "Alternate Intimacies," pages 42–44).

As you think about these questions, there are a few points to keep in mind. First, once the early newlywed period is over, you may realize that you each have differing levels of desire and need for intimacy. This type of disparity is experienced by many couples and requires communication and negotiation to keep both of you feeling comfortable. For example, if one of you is content with having sexual intercourse once a month and the other would like to have sex every night that you're halachically permitted to do so, this issue can easily escalate into a source of tension, with both of you feeling hurt and frustrated. While an open conversation on this issue is not easy, it is crucial for a couple to begin these discussions sooner rather than later, enabling them to develop a mutually satisfying solution. One example could be the flexible use of time; a person who is too tired to consider intimacy at night might feel very different early in the morning or at another more convenient time of day.

Another point is that physical intimacy has no absolute fixed dosage. Sexual frequency changes over the course of a couple's marriage and is affected by many factors, including physical issues (such as pregnancy, childbirth, or illness), emotional issues (such as grief or anxiety), relationship issues (such as tensions or problems in the broader marriage relationship), the general busyness of life as your family grows, and work or financial stresses. Almost every factor that affects your life will affect your sexual life as well. Some life experiences may lead to a decrease in sexual desire, which is not necessarily a sign of a problem in the relationship, but rather is a reflection of the difficult time that either spouse is currently experiencing. Even without sad or negative events emerging in your lives, positive events – such as pregnancy or the birth of a child – may have a similar impact on the sexual relationship (for more about pregnancy and childbirth, see pages 48–53).

Frustration with *Niddah*

> THEY ASK: *We've been married for around six months and every time we're in* niddah *we both feel so depressed. It's frustrating to come home at the end of a long day and not even be able to give each other a hug.* Baruch Hashem *we have a great relationship and try to express our love for each other even during* niddah, *but sometimes we both end up feeling alone and rejected. Is there anything we can do to cope?*

Almost all religious couples struggle with *niddah* at some point in their relationship. Especially in the beginning of your marriage, when you're still adjusting to the newness of everything, *niddah* can be a recurring source of stress. The good news is that it does get better with time, especially if you're willing to work at it. Though each couple is different, here are some suggestions that might help.

- Try to determine when each of you is most susceptible to feeling alone and rejected – is it before you go to bed, when you wake up in the morning, when you come home from work? These are great times to verbally express affection and understanding for each other.

- Find ways of expressing your affection that don't involve touch: encourage each other to articulate your feelings, maybe leave little notes around the house or send text messages to show that you are still thinking of each other.

- Don't stop spending time together in your efforts to avoid physical contact. Avoiding each other during *niddah* is a mistake that some young couples make – it may send a message to your spouse that you are only able to interact with each other in a physical way. *Niddah* is a time to deepen your nonphysical avenues of communication and relationship.

- Get out of the apartment: some couples find that they're more likely to feel tension, conflict, or hopelessness during *niddah* when they stay home. Getting out for a change of scenery can do wonders for alleviating this stress. Whether you go out for dinner, go for a walk around the block, or go somewhere more adventurous, just getting outside may do you both good.

- While until now we've offered suggestions as to what you can do as a couple when in *niddah*, it's also important to find time for yourselves as individuals during this period. In the newlywed stage, you may find that in adjusting to marriage and getting to know each other, you have not been able to spend as much time as usual on your own pursuits or seeing your friends: *niddah* is a good time for you each to do things you don't generally do together.

Intimacy in Someone Else's Home

THEY ASK: We've been married for almost a year, and we find ourselves spending most Shabbosim away from home, either at one of our parents' houses or with friends. We both feel uncomfortable being intimate when we're staying in someone else's house, and our attempts at sexual intercourse there just don't seem to work. What can we do?

It's difficult for many couples to let their guard down and be intimate in either their parents' or their in-laws' home – and for sex to be good, letting your guard down is essential. In friends' homes as well it can be hard to relax, especially if you're staying in close quarters and don't have the same amount of privacy that you do in your own home. Be guided by your feelings; it's definitely legitimate for you to decide as a couple that you simply won't have intercourse when visiting with friends or family.

If Shabbos has become a time for going away, then you need to work to find other times during the week when you both feel more comfortable being sexual with each other, or else start spending Shabbos together in your own home. Maybe making love when you come home from your Shabbos travels feels right; or maybe making love before you go away works for you; or maybe you just want to be open to the spontaneity of the moment – the possibilities are all there for you to enjoy. Just because Shabbos isn't the day that works best now doesn't mean that you can't have a positive sex life during the rest of the week.

External Pressures Affecting Your Sex Life

THEY ASK: We've been married for almost a year and have had some wonderful times exploring our sexuality. However, our lease is up and we need to move by next month, and we haven't been able to find a new apartment – and the stress is getting to both of us to the point that it's diminishing our desire and ability to have sex. What can we do?

THEY ASK: My husband lost his job a few weeks ago. Since then he just hasn't been interested in being intimate and has avoided my advances – sex has always been a positive part of our marriage but now I don't know what to do.

THEY ASK: My wife's sister suddenly passed away six months ago and since then my wife has been completely absorbed in her grief and uninterested in sex. Will this ever go away?

These questions emphasize that physical intimacy is a part of life and can't be isolated from the totality of your existence. Work problems, financial crises, apartment woes, grief, and exhaustion all can inhibit a person's desire and enjoyment of sex. Not everyone responds the same way to these circumstances, and some may even specifically turn to sex in times of crisis in order to find love and security. If your sexual life has been positive and enjoyable before, then it's important to understand that once the external crisis clears up, your intimate life will likely return to its regular rhythm.

During this time it is particularly advisable to communicate openly and to find ways to stay close as a couple – you need to stick together to get through this crisis, and it's important that you talk about the range of feelings that you are experiencing (in the sexual realm and beyond).

It's also helpful that you not lose sight of alternate forms of physical intimacy. Sometimes when sexual intercourse is not desired by either of you, something more supportive and gentle can really bring you added closeness. Hugs and kisses can offer both comfort and love, and snuggling under the covers together can help you temporarily escape from your troubles!

Some Parting Thoughts

As we end this work, there are a few points that we want to reiterate. No matter how much we may try to shield ourselves from it, popular culture plays a huge role in our expectations. Despite what you might have absorbed from movies, TV, or other media, it's important to realize that real-life sex is not necessarily a smooth and seamless experience, so adjust your expectations accordingly. The newlywed stage is unique in its wonder and newness and also in its challenges. Experience this special part of your lives together as a couple and take the time to invest in your sexual relationship now. Building a strong foundation in this area will benefit your marriage for years to come. With that in mind, don't hesitate to contact a sexual health professional to help you with any uncertainty and guide you to a better place.

Marriage is a journey with multiple phases. Intimacy too will have different meanings at various stages in your lives. Sex at the beginning of a marriage differs from sex while raising young children, and both of these differ from sex when your children have left the house and you are grandparents. In each stage, sex can find its place as part of your broader relationship. There will be times in your life when sex is a more intense part of your marital intimacy and times when it may be less intense. This is perfectly normal. This book was designed to help you through some of the initial issues that you may face in your physical and emotional relationship. As time goes by, new challenges may take the place of earlier ones and you will find additional resources to draw upon.

The verse in Proverbs (3:6) – "בכל דרכיך דעהו, in all your ways know Him" – instructs us that in every aspect of our lives we should seek

HaKadosh Baruch Hu. There is no action that is too mundane within which to find Godliness. This is especially true of the sexual relationship, which has the potential for truly being a space of holiness. We hope and pray that through deepening your connection with each other physically, emotionally, and sexually, you also come to a deeper connection with *Hashem* and merit building together a *bayis ne'eman b'Yisrael*.

This work is the first of its kind and therefore your feedback is especially important to us. If you have any comments or questions, please contact us at etleehov.intimacy@gmail.com.

Resources

Some of you may wish further information on the topics covered in these pages. Although the lack of accurate sexual material for religious couples was one of the main factors that motivated our writing this book, we have not been able to include everything, and so we offer you this list. Because these resources were not prepared with a religious audience in mind, many of them have content that is not relevant or appropriate for you. Please take this into account before using any of this material.

For Couples

Guide to Getting It On
Paul Joannides
Goofy Foot Press (2009)
Though this book uses slang and "street language," no other book can compete with its comprehensiveness, and its wit sets a comfortable tone.

What Your Mother Never Told You about S-E-X
Hilda Hutcherson, MD
Perigee Books (2003)
This book has a nice tone, uses minimal slang, and has basic information about male and female anatomy, and different forms of giving and receiving sexual pleasure throughout the lifespan.

The Joy of Sex: The Timeless Guide to Lovemaking, Ultimate Revised Edition
Alex Comfort and Susan Quilliam
Crown Publishers (2009)
This new edition has been almost entirely rewritten to make it consistent with recent research and more focused on mutual enjoyment.

The Sex-Starved Marriage: A Couple's Guide to Boosting Their Marriage Libido
Michele Weiner-Davis
Simon and Schuster (2003)
Written in a pleasant, matter-of-fact style, this book offers a range of practical advice to help couples rekindle their sexual desire.

The Ultimate Guide to Sex and Disability: For All of Us Who Live with Disabilities, Chronic Pain, and Illness
Miriam Kaufman, MD, Cory Silverberg, and Fran Odette
Cleis Press (2007)
This is an excellent, positively-toned resource for those coping with physical disabilities that may have an impact on sexual desire and behaviors.

Go Ask Alice! This internet resource, produced by a division of Health Services at Columbia University, provides answers to thousands of questions about sex and sexuality.
www.goaskalice.com

The Sexuality Information and Education Council of the United States (SIECUS) provides up-to-date sexuality information through publications, websites, and other resources.
www.siecus.org

The American Association of Sexuality Educators, Counselors, and Therapists (AASECT) provides certification for sexual therapy, counseling, and education. This is a great site for locating certified sex therapists in your area worldwide, as well as downloading information on sexuality.
www.aasect.org

Natural Contours, a company known for reliability, manufactures and sells vibrators that are ergonomically engineered to fit the curves of a woman's body.
www.natural-contours.com

Good Vibrations is a reputable website, which has been around for over thirty years, for purchasing all types of sexual items (lubricant, vibrators, etc.).
www.goodvibes.com

For Women

I Love Female Orgasm
Dorian Solot and Marshall Miller
Da Capo Press (2007)
This is an excellent book on female orgasm, written in a comfortable, friendly, and instructive tone.

The Elusive Orgasm: A Woman's Guide to Why She Can't and How She Can Orgasm
Vivienne Cass, PhD
Da Capo Press (2007)
A bit more technical with lots of helpful diagrams.

A Woman's Guide to Overcoming Sexual Fear and Pain
Aurelie J. Goodwin, EdD, and Marc E. Agronin

New Harbinger Publications (1997)
This gentle guide uses clinical examples and women's personal accounts to help achieve sexual satisfaction, and offers exercises and suggestions for specific disorders.

Private Pain: It's About Life, Not Just Sex; Understanding Vaginismus and Dyspareunia
Ditza Katz, PT, PhD, and Ross Lynn Tabisel, LCSW, PhD
Katz-Tabi Publications (2005)
Written by observant women, this book does a great job legitimizing the feelings of women who suffer from painful intercourse, and gives practical advice and resources on how to cope with it.

Our Bodies, Ourselves: A New Edition for a New Era
Boston Women's Health Book Collective
Touchstone (2005)
This book, first written in the 1960s, contains valuable information for women on women's health and sexual issues throughout the lifespan, as well as navigating the American health care system.

The Women's Sexual Health Foundation (TWSHF) provides a multidisciplinary approach to the treatment of sexual health issues.
www.twshf.org

The National Institutes of Health maintains an excellent source of health information for women.
www.womenshealth.com

For Men

Unfortunately, there are far fewer quality resources targeted specifically at male sexuality.

The New Male Sexuality
Dr. Bernie Zilbergeld
Bantam Books (1999)
An excellent overview of men's sexual health concerns, this book offers options for coping with sexual dysfunctions.

The National Institutes of Health makes available an excellent source of health information for men.
http://www.nlm.nih.gov/medlineplus/menshealth.html

About the Authors

Jennie Rosenfeld holds a PhD in English from the City University of New York Graduate Center, and has done research on contemporary Modern Orthodox sexual ethics. Previously, she served as the cofounder and director of Tzelem, a Special Project of Yeshiva University, whose goal was to bring more sexual education resources to different constituents within the Orthodox community.

David S. Ribner earned his *smichah* (ordination) and MSW degree from Yeshiva University and his doctorate from Columbia University. He is the founder and director of the Sex Therapy Training Program, School of Social Work, Bar-Ilan University, and is certified as a sex therapist in Israel and the United States. He is in private practice as a sex and marital therapist in Jerusalem and writes and lectures extensively on Judaism and sexuality.